YOGA IS A MANTRA

May God's great name be glorified and sanctified throughout the world He has created . . .

Om

YOGA IS A MANTRA
A Tool to Discover One's Self

LALIT K. KILAM

Om Mani Padme Hum!

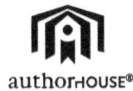

authorHOUSE®

AuthorHouse™
1663 Liberty Drive
Bloomington, IN 47403
www.authorhouse.com
Phone: 1-800-839-8640

Published by AuthorHouse 2/28/2012

ISBN: 978-1-4685-3983-7 (sc)
ISBN: 978-1-4685-3982-0 (hc)
ISBN: 978-1-4685-3981-3 (ebk)

Library of Congress Control Number: 2012900113

CONTENTS

CONTENTS

ACKNOWLEDGMENTS

I express my sincere gratitude and love to Dr. Peter K. Raina and Halina, to my brother Dr. S. K. Kilam, and Janice and Ashwani Kilam. Support of the family is always of a great importance to me.

I extend my gratefulness to Mr. Nehru and Krishna Didi for always being there for me.

I am very grateful to all my teachers who taught me all along. Without their personal guidance, I would not have engaged in the natural sciences and in the living tradition of yoga or its practical dimensions, philosophy, and implications in daily life.

Hikaru-san, with her grace, who is always kinder than the kindest, made the writing of this work a joyous task. I deeply thank her.

I owe a lot to my parents, who have always given me their blessings. I thank all my dear friends from various learning schools for their thoughts and discussions of philosophy with me.

I would like to thank and I am obliged to all the beautiful people whom I met on streets, in cafés, and in various bookshops while I was working on this book. Their smiles, more than anything else, made me realize an ability to rise above any situation.

Last yet not least, I express my thanks to my publisher, editor Ms. Sue Ducharme, Mr. Zack DePew, and all the staff for their most valuable contribution to make this work a complete success. I express my sincere thanks to Ms. Margaret Michna for her valuable and warm support. My great regards to Mr. Marcus Reeves for his kind suggestions. My heart goes out to thank Ms. Kathryn E. Schwoerer for her continued support from the first day in every aspect of making this volume a finished product.

With prayers

Eng. **Lalit Kilam**

CHAPTER I

Yoga a means for the existence of man

The world in which we exist . . . will pass away, burnt up in the fire of its own hot passions; and from its ashes will spring a new and younger world, but full of fresh hope, with the light of morning in its eyes.

Bernard Russell

The first premise of all human history is the existence of the human race. The human race distinguishes itself from animals by its consciousness, beliefs, values, religious faith, and much more. Since early history, humans have been preoccupied in finding satisfactory answers to the question of their existence.

In the early stages of civilization many tribes worshipped ghosts, tribal gods, demons, and the spirits of their forefathers; even today a few tribes might follow such practices. Why do they do this? Because, deep down, they feel that in some unknown way these beings are greater and more powerful and limit mankind in some mysterious ways. Therefore, they seek to propitiate these beings, to prevent them from interfering with them. They also seek to win favors from these beings, in the form of good fortunes, wealth, et cetera. Historically, we human beings expect miracles to take place, thereby solving all our earthly problems. This expectation never leaves us. However we say it, we are all hoping for unbelievable and extraordinary events to happen in our lives. According to Max Muller, religion enables man to apprehend the infinite, under different names and varying guises. "Religion is belief in God."

Religion and mysticism live a world of faith and vision, while science and philosophy live in a world of verified facts. When a person dies, it is said, "You cannot take wealth, family, or possessions with you. But there is something very important that you can take with you: your accumulated virtues wisdom, and karma. All else is left behind. The only thing that remains is the karma that we have accumulated through our actions, words, and thoughts.

In the beginning God created the heavens and earth. He created humankind in his image according to his likeness. He cannot be seen with the human eye, nor comprehended by speech. He can only be attained by with a special comprehension of the positive knowledge's given to us; mainly in a form of revelation or otherwise and by our actions and the karmas we do.

Unfortunately a great human tradition has been running away from the Creator who made possible the miracle of life so that we exist. Adam hid in the Garden of Eden. Moses tried to substitute his brother. Jonah jumped a boat and was swallowed by whale.

According to a philosophy of Plato, only deeply virtuous people can actually attain positive knowledge of the truth and achieve genuine understanding of God. Plato believes that there are different kinds of desires, if thought is given to this logical analysis; these are energies present in our subjective aspect, driving us to do our present karmas and damning the nobleness of thought, word, and deed. On the basis of Plato's philosophy of desire: (1) appetitive desires, for food, drink, sex, and the money with which to acquire them; (2) spiritual desire for honor, victory, and a good reputation; and (3) rational desire for knowledge and truth. These desires are located in different parts of the soul that determine man's character. He is a money-lover if he is ruled by appetite, an honor-lover if he is ruled by the spiritual part of his soul, and a wisdom-lover, or a philosopher, if his soul is ruled by its rational part. In other words, the concept of God is naturally dependent on what we want from our existence, and what we strive for in our lives defines the purpose of living and our existence. Pure knowledge is a guide for having a conversation with God; perhaps it is the fountainhead of our belief system and the karmas/deeds we do in day-to-day life. It is not significant how a human being has this conversation with God, but what is indeed important is to express our thankfulness to God that he is the Creator. He is the one who gave us life to exist. The moment we sense that there is something more to life than having an appetite or desire, we will spontaneously start praying to Him. Considering this, the subjective aspect of human life becomes a priority in our civilization, not only from a technological or sociopolitical point of view, but also in simply realizing that we are individual entities responsible for our own actions and inactions and that we exist. A broader study of human behavior started first at one of the philosophical schools in Europe. Plato offered this idea first.

Human history also confirms that our subjective aspect is comprised of the science of mathematics and linguistics; great astrologers like Copernicus and many other theorists stressed the subjective aspect of a human being. Even in recent times, a Persian astrologer expressed *Her Kamale Ra Zawale; Her Zawale Ra Kamale*; mainly the priority of the subjective aspect.

All of this is presently being treated as stories, theories, and long-forgotten metaphysical problems, though they are based on all the sciences provided to us with which we operate in our daily lives, knowingly or unknowingly.

Study of all the existing knowledge in any field at modern educational institutions no doubt makes us only gurus or idlers, an idea widely advanced by Sir George Bernard Shaw in his great writings.

A mindful student educating himself will never become a guru because of his scholarship and humbleness at academia, where access to vast and noble resources is not limited to the resources in a *bibliothek*. Academia is equipped with practical and sacred tools; may their influence inspire us to breathe love into our hearts. It will indeed bring grace to the soul.

Students will not only learn about the energy systems governing our internal and external realms created by God, but also how to harmonize these energies within themselves and fellow students and become able to define the basis of belief, consciousness, and karmas/actions done knowingly or unknowingly. Students will also learn to be thankful to the Lord, for he created us to exist; by his scholarship he will always learn the new science and knowledge. He will keep himself always in his presence; he will pray for the right comprehension of the only word which exists . . . the Lord.

Having an attitude to learn makes a more homogeneous society in the world we inhabit today. As written by Sir Winston Churchill, "Let us remember only so much of the past as will make us creative for the future."

PRAYERS

I have been driven many times to my knees by the overwhelming conviction that I had nowhere else to go. My own wisdom, and that of all about me, seemed insufficient for the day.—*Abraham Lincoln*

Father in heaven, when the thought of you wakes in our hearts, let it not wake like a frightened bird that flies about in dismay, but like a child waking from its sleep with a heavenly smile.—*Soren Kierkegaard*

God is the cause of all things, which are in him.—*Benedict Spinoza*

It is thoroughly necessary to be convinced of God's existence; it is not quite so necessary that one should demonstrate it.—*Immanuel Kant*

The savour of wandering in the ocean of deathless life has rid me of all my asking; as the tree is in the seed, so all diseases are in this asking.—*Kabir*

On this road with no traveler Autumn night falls.—*Matsuo Basho*

God sends things down on us as a warning so that we may ponder and change our ways. The merciful Lord seeks us to do good deeds and also says: urge one another to steadfastness and compassion.

We exist because God wants us to exist. We are made by God and for God. Life will make sense only when we understand that otherwise life will not make any sense. We discover our origin, our identity, the purpose of our life, its meaning and significance only in God. He can only be attained by the positive knowledge of what we believe in and by our actions and karmas. Knowledge we could never attain, reminding us what we are, may be attainable by acknowledging the higher powers and a higher life, which we may achieve also by being moral and virtuous.

Blessed are the pure in heart, for they shall see God. (Matthew 5:8)

The same idea was expressed by a Sufi poet, Jalal-uddin Rumi, in terms of a scientific metaphor: "The astrolable of the mysteries of God is love."

There is an indivisible unity between karma and dharma, as also said in one of the Buddhist mantras: Om Mani Padme Hum. Dharma determines our true essence: morality, righteousness, ethics, compassion, and a lawful order of the universe. Human pursuit is to seek dharma (i.e., to transform our body, thought, and word into an exalted Buddha). We can reach this state also by practicing yoga is a mantra in our daily life. It is something you naturally are, your internal realm. It is not something you have to train for or a skill you want to add. It is just a reminder to return home. Kashmiri Yoga practice is to return home to what is natural to you (i.c., freedom of thought).

Yoga as a mantra is a method of awareness. A seeker of the Eastern sun, a yogi delves into consciousness itself, ignoring all the negative influences surrounding him at that moment. He unites his thought, word, and body, hoping to be in the plane which is beyond all knowledge, that point where subject and object no longer exist.

An ancient mystic known as the soul of Kashmir, Lalla Ded used to say, "I, Lalla, entered through the garden-gate of my soul; There, o Joy! I found the Yoga Shiva united with Shakti. Overwhelmed, I got immersed in the lake of Nectar. Even though alive or dead, what can existence do unto me?"

In many creative activities, we are faced with choices and are not sure of the correct approach. It is just like a car stuck in the sand; the wheels are moving, but the vehicle stays still. According to the philosophy of Kant, a human being can differentiate between the empirical realm and the non-empirical, on the basis of reason. Consciousness, like language, arises from needs in the empirical realm, which is governed by the scientific laws, while the non-empirical realm is governed by universal, cosmic laws. In the non-empirical realm, body moments and the choices we make are governed by the cosmic laws. In dharma/karma, one of the cosmic laws is the human law, which depends on the evolution of our bodies, thoughts, and language defined in this work as a sacred code. Yoga is a mantra protects one's existence in whatever situation one is in.

Yoga as a mantra, the sacred code, is a part of human consciousness given to us at the time of birth by the mysterious ways of God. To formulate an algorithm based on this metaphysical hypothesis and to reach certain positive results in the form of enlightenment by the practices/abhyasa of any of the sacred tools provided to us by the Lord. Yoga is a mantra, and its practices, known as Sadhna, is one of the tools. Practicing yoga asanas, pranayama, and meditation with a vision toward the infinite and mindfulness toward all the sacred directions and places, like Ganga, Ka'ba, or an ancient cathedral, develops in us the meaning of our universal existence. This approach leads us to the path of morality, righteousness, compassion, and love and to a virtuous living. According to some prominent philosophies, sufferings (duhkha) are with us since the creation, phenomenal or internal. In a human being they arise because of our cravings and desires for everything material and mental. According to the philosophy of yoga, a path of disinterested action and karma also removes the duhkha, or sufferings.

As Dostoevski said: "There is only one thing that I dread; not to be worthy of my sufferings."

According to the philosophy of Buddha the main cause of sufferings is *mara*. If we differentiate ourselves from any other animate or inanimate being we could avoid it by our karmas, or actions, which cause the entire cycle of transmigration that governs our existence.

The positive and negative actions of a human being cause karmas. Vedas have written about the karmic cycle state, "If an individual sows goodness, he will reap goodness; if one sows evil, he will reap evil." Karma is a principle that governs the energies and the direction of our thoughts, words, bodies, and deeds as embodied in our sacred code.

We as individual entities are, in a way, our karmas. The current Advanced Cybernatical Society or considering the history of ancient river valley civilizations does it have any positive effect on our internal conditioning/subjective aspect of a man. Perhaps not *mara*, which no doubt in this work also a part of the internal human conditioning just as a cloud which has made our Sun hazy leading us to a plane of existence where there is no Word as belief. Nevertheless not taking into consideration the existence of thought and the meditative practices explained by a young Lama Christie McNally, sadly to say we will be at the same stage of evolution where Charles Darwin started.

"You have heard that it was said, 'you shall love your neighbor and hate your enemy.' But I say to you, Love your enemies and pray for those who persecute you, so that you may be children of your Father in heaven; for he makes his sun rise on the evil and on the good, and sends rain on the righteous and on the unrighteous. For if you love those who love you, what reward do you have? Do not even the tax collectors do the same? And if you greet only your brothers and sisters, what more are you doing than others? Do not even the Gentiles do the same? Be perfect, therefore, as your heavenly Father is perfect." (Matthew 5:24).

"A man is created to work and be judged. He should therefore seek to do good deeds rather than indulge in arrogance and wastefulness." (The Qur'an 90:20)

"Thou art Mother, Thou art Father, Thou art Kinsman, Thou art Friend, Thou art Knowledge, Thou art Wealth, Thou art my all, O Lord of Lords." (The Gita)

There is God's grace for every human being because he knows what is happening in his creation; He sends always his archangel as a messenger between the Heaven and Earth at the time when a man deviates from the thought why he exists on this earth.

Philosopher Benedict Spinoza mainly studied mathematics and linguistics, he said that God exists and is infinite and a perfect being. But if God is infinite then he cannot have limits, cannot have boundaries, and if he had them, then he would be finite. So Spinoza's philosophy says that there cannot be anything that God is not.

He, the Lord God, the absolute, created many sacred tools for human beings, including yoga as a mantra. Through the practice of yoga as a mantra in daily life, our karmas will acquire the altruistic intention to become enlightened; it will open the storehouse of our latent wisdom, which will bring grace to our soul in the form of freedom of thought compassion.

BODY

According to the philosophy of yoga, the human body is divided into three categories, namely the physical, subtle or astral, and causal. The combinations of the five great elements, fire, water, earth, space, and air, and their combinations make the structure of our body as defined in Ayurveda. These elements exist within us and in everything. If the percentage of the combinations of these elements is known, we can do better to preserve our health by doing appropriate yoga asanas. These elements, or energies, define our body moments and control our movements to do positive Karma's.

WORDS OR SPEECH

Speech is the only means to convey and communicate. It also is based on sounds, music, et cetera. Grace and gracelessness follow good or bad rhythm. Good rhythm follows good words and vice versa, which is the same for harmony and disharmony.

In the *Descent of Man*, Darwin wrote that language "has justly been considered as one of the chief distinctions between man and the lower animals." There are four stages in the manifestation of verbal expressions. Speech is not only the means to convey ideas; it is also a way to comprehend ideas based on just the sounds. The Egyptians were the first people to develop a system of writing, at almost the same time as the Sumerians. The script was an independent one; it began as picture writing and was later combined with pictographs. This was called sacred carvings. Most of the writing was done on fine paper made from papyrus. A finer form of speech that serves as a medium for thinking and understanding, through which a human being forms definite and indefinite ideas about words and their meanings, is called as mental speech. It is the reflection of our internal realm taking the form of ideas. There is still finer level of speech, far subtler in character, which resides in the innermost part of our being. Beyond this is supreme speech, or transcendental speech. Transcendental speech consists of pure awareness of our consciousness.

Yoga is a mantra is also classified as an art; mindfulness toward the subjective aspect and practicing this art will not only remove the existing unfavorable linguistic conditions but also decondition our internal existing conditions through the practice of yoga asanas and by having an attitude toward a living philosophy:

A home for one . . . A home for all.

It will make a difference in our existence.

CHAPTER II

The Vedic Philosophy and Yoga

VEDIC PHILOSOPHY

Vedas are knowledge. Its aim is to help find solutions to the mystery of all human existence. A great Western scholar Max Muller used to say that Rig Veda had a great formative influence in his life. Some philosophers have varied opinions about the study of Vedic literature, as the solutions presented are diverse and many. Some consider it to be religion and mysticism, others a theology; for others it is soteriology, or theology based on salvation. For yet others it is the rudiments of scientific teachings. Vedanta is a pure philosophy; it seeks not the imaginary or abstract, but a verifiable and true explanation for existence. The fundamental principle of Vedanta is oneness, and that oneness is on the highest spiritual plane. There is one life, which exists; one spirit, one truth, and one reality. What distinguishes Vedanta from all other human pursuits is that it does not rest till it attains the ultimate goal of universal freedom by doing away with all sorrows. This it does by probing into the mysteries of existence. This might be difficult; not everyone will be able to attain the ultimate truth.

Vedas are broadly divided into two parts, namely:

1) Karma-Kanda
2) Janana-Kanda

Karma-Kanda is devoted to the work portion and is recommended before the beginning of the spiritual portion. The Janana-Kanda is devoted to the knowledge portion of the teachings of the Upanishads.

1) The Karma-Kanda may further be roughly divided into three parts:

1. The Mantras, or hymns, are sung in adoration of the gods. The Samhitas of Rig Vedas is a collection of hymns and songs, handed down by the ancestors. They had been first used in adoration of the father of Heaven, of sun, of Dawn, and of Agni, the god of fire. These are mostly nature gods. These are prayers for health, wealth, long life, victory in the battle field, and freedom from the bonds of sins committed.

2. The Brahmanas are written as prose describing the sacrificial rites, including precepts, charities, and religious duties. Sacrificial rites and treatises on their significance are performed by Brahmins. This is when the heart becomes purified by the performance of sacrifices and charities that enhances the desire for knowledge.

3. The Aranyakas, or forest treaties, supplant the external rituals with symbolic meditations. The knowledge found here is not an end in itself, but enables one to perform the actions that gain an end. The main idea of Karma-Kanda consists of the duties of man, the duties of the householder, the duties of the recluse, and the various duties in different stages of the life cycle.

VEDIC CONCEPT OF GOD

In many Vedic hymns, the gods are represented as the controlling and presiding powers behind natural phenomena. The Vedic Rishi saw the sun, Moon, Sea, Water, Earth, Fire, and Sky as divine entities and not as integrated parts of nature. These forces of nature are unpredictable and have an amazing power at their command. Very often the same characteristics are attributed to the various deities, or divas.

The Aryans worshipped these forces as gods and called them as Divas, or Devis, which means "The Giver," as they give the most important forces for the survival of a man. Man considered them as human beings in thoughts and form. Therefore, like human beings, they were born from a superior God. Thus eventually all these Divas became related to each other. They also thought like human beings, suffered from human weaknesses, and discussed and debated issues like man; they can be pleased in the way we please another human being. In the initial phase of the Vedic era, prayer was sufficient to please the gods. Later on gods became more demanding and required sacrifices and offerings for their pleasure.

Almost every temple represents the nature deities. The holy names of gods in Vedas are according to their nature, knowledge, and deeds. Gods create, preserve, destroy, and control the universe. Therefore those names are eternal and countless.

For Vedic man, the truth, Rta, has to be obeyed and appeased by means of sacrificial celebrations. The Aryans and Rishi worshipped Yajna as Divas and Devis with Rig Vedic mantras, which were masked with symbols and symbolic words. Secrecy was observed, restoring to double meaning a device possible in the Sanskrit language. Rishi composed the mantras as a means of spiritual progress for himself and for others. It rose from his consciousness and became a power of his mind and also a source of self-expression.

Prayers and praise to the gods were meant to induce them to shower on the sacrifices material blessings, such as plenty of cows, horses, fighting men, sons, food, wealth of all kinds, protection, victory in battle, bringing down rain from the heavens, or recovering the sun from the clouds and from the grip of night.

The word for *cow* meant a ray of light. By this formulation the seers, or the Rishis, meant truth, light, and knowledge, which were the rays of the Sun God. By *plenty of horses*, the Rishis meant spiritual strength or the force of tapasya/penance.

SURYA, GOD OF LIGHT

Surya is the god of light and a symbol of self in the Vedic text. It is the only visible form of God that can be seen every day. Surya is also known as Surya Narayana and is acknowledged as one of the eight forms of Lord Shiva. It is believed that Surya has been worshipped since time immemorial to receive the kind blessings of God. A known mode of worship to the Sun God is the Surya Namaskara, or the Sun Salutation.

About ten hymns are addressed to Surya in Rig Veda. Surya is also spoken as a wheel (chakra) representing the eight energy centers in the human body. The Gayatri-Mantra frequently recited to praise the Surya comes from Rig Veda:

Om Bhur-Bhuvah-Svah
Tat-Savitur-Varenyam
Bhargo-Devasya-Dhimahi
Dhiyo-Yo-Nah-Pracodayat

Having realized the light in the sun is the dispeller of ignorance and is the same as the light within our hearts, and thus having realized the light that is higher than the other lights, we attain the sun, the light that is the best of all lights, brightest among the lights.

AGNI, GOD OF FIRE

Agni is one of the most important Vedic gods. He is the god of fire, lightning, and the sun, the messenger of gods, the acceptor of sacrifices. The sacrifices made to Agni go to the deities, because Agni is messenger from and to other gods.

Agni is the first word of the first hymn in the Rig Veda. He is the supreme Brahmin of the religious ceremonies and duties, signified as a messenger. Agni is the mystery of our birth and death.

He is the mediator between God and worshippers who offer their oblations and sacrifices, the outgoing into incoming breath and the incoming into outgoing; retaining the breath, constantly practicing the regulation of the vital energy (prana). The senses are thus attenuated and are merged as unified prana as an act of sacrifice. The individual soul is symbolized by fire, meaning the inner guide. Agni is the spiritual consciousness that builds from within; it contains the essence, the source, of who we are and all that we can become.

VAYU GOD OF WIND

Vayu is the great Vedic personification of wind. His other names are Vatam, Pavana, or Prana.

The Sanskrit word *vata* means blown: Vayu: blower, and prana: breathing; that is, the breath of life, or the deity of Life. There are five deities of Vayu: Prna; Apana; Vyana; Udana, and Samana. These are the vital breath that controls life. It is the basis of all life. Inside our bodies, he works as the five vital airs; Vayu is the place where everything merges. When fire goes out, it merges into air. When the sun sets, it merges into air. When the moon sets, it merges into air. Vayu, the external air, is the place of merger; it swallows everything.

The mantra frequently recited to praise Vayu comes from Rig Veda:

> Oh! Beautiful Vayu, god of the wind, come, for the libations of the juice of the Soma, or moon plant, have been prepared. The plant was gathered by moonlight on certain mountains, stripped of its leaves, and then carried to the place of sacrifice. The stalks have been crushed by the Brahmin and sprinkled with water and placed on a sieve, and after further pressure the juice trickled into a vessel, and after which it was mixed with flour, et cetera and made to ferment, and then offered in libations to the gods or drunk by Brahmins. Oh! Vayu, drink of them, hear our invocations.

PRITHVI, GOD OF EARTH

In the Rig Veda, earth and sky are frequently addressed in the dual, indicating the idea of two complementary half-shells. Prithvi is also called Dharti, or earth, meaning that which holds everything. Earth is the only element linked to all the five senses—taste; sound; touch; smell; and sight—and thus exerts the maximum influence on us. One can touch earth and smell it too. There are two types of earth: eternal, which is in the form of an atom, and perishable, which exists in the form of Karya, or work. Our body and sense organs are the earth, which as a whole is in the shape of Jiva, or matter, which is perishable. But the elements of atoms are eternal; after death we may bury or burn the body, but all the atoms come back to their original eternal form. So our body and its Karya, or work, are perishable but the atoms remain which are eternal. God is in the earth; hence, the people worship the god of earth and receive divine blessings.

JAL, GOD OF WATER

Oh! God of water, whatever sin has been found in me and all the evils in me or whatever I have knowingly done wrong, or cursed the holy men or uttered untruth, take it away from me.—Rig Veda

Cosmically, Apah are the waters of space, out of which the universe is produced. The waters assume different forms on this earth: the atmosphere, the sky, mountains, gods and humans, beasts and birds, grass and trees, animals and worms, flies and ants. Apah is all these forms.

Waters are celestial and terrestrial, and the sea is their goal. They abide where the gods dwell. They are mothers and as such produce Agni. They give their auspicious fluid, like loving mothers. They purify sins. They even cleanse moral guilt, the sins of violence, cursing, and lying. They also bestow remedies, health, wealth, strength, long life, and immortality.

The celestial waters are identified with heavenly Soma, for Indra, the Vedic deity. Water has been an object of worship from time immemorial. Water represents non-manifested substratum from which all manifestations arise.

AKASHA, GOD OF SKY

Akasha is a Sanskrit word meaning ether. Akasha is infinite and limitless. It is related to our sense of hearing. Ether is a material that fills the regions of the universe above the terrestrial sphere. In Greek mythology ether means pure, fresh air or clear sky, where the gods live and which they breathe. Ether is unique; it has only one characteristic, which is that it is eternal. It is the carrier of sound, be it man-made or otherwise. It attracted the attention of great sages in the form of divine sound that is heard by the sages of higher order. Ether, time, and space are eternal. OM is a symbol of form, as well as sound, which is the manifestation of spiritual power.

VEDIC YOGA: THE STRUCTURE OF KASHMIRI YOGA

The specific power of the mantra is to invoke the gods by inner sacrifice and offer them the gifts of sacrifice. God is one, but Rishis who were learned in Vedas uttered so many names for one god: Agni, Vayu, Prithvi, Sky, sun, and Water. The holy names of God in Vedas are according to the nature, knowledge, and deeds of almighty God. And therefore those names are eternal and countless. Often the deities are assigned to a backseat in the new philosophical age, with the result that there is less understanding of the deities and the important role they play in the spiritual growth and less conscious understanding regarding deities. These deities represent common cosmic principles, not just the mystical but also the practical applications of the life principle. Vedic Yoga is filled with deities, offering a variety of techniques depending on the consciousness and ability of the practitioner.

Vedic Yoga, or Kashmiri Yoga, does not include the postures commonly associated with yoga. It does include mudras for mantra, pranayama, and meditation itself. It includes the sun and the moon of the Hatha Yoga tradition. It contains wisdom, representing Jnana Yoga. Bhakti Yoga also includes Vedas and reverence for deities. For a novice, these Vedic deities provide access into deeper regions of the mind, resulting in expanded awareness and mental performance. From the view point of yoga traditions, it is impossible to separate yoga from Vedic deities, as they represent the universal force of creation and transformation.

Yoga Is a Mantra involves developing Mantra Shakti, the power of mantra, through which the mantra becomes alive as a tool of transformation in the mind. From this arises mantric insight, through which the inner meaning of the mantra can be grasped, thereby linking us with the divine laws.

Vedic Yoga forms the structure of Kashmiri Yoga, also known as Shambavopaya, which is at the highest and most subtle quantum energetic plane—the most direct and quickest path to yoga is a mantra, but surely the most difficult to master.

In the mystical union of Shiva and Shakti, Shiva is unchanging consciousness and Shakti is its unchanging power; Shiva is able to function only when united with his Shakti. Otherwise he is inert. It originated in the mountainous region of Kashmir for the betterment of humankind, having no boundaries whatsoever, and is known as the Pratyabhina system. Consciousness, though it moves in differentiated states of its own existence, is free, but it never falls from its internal realm or its true nature.

In order to succeed, a student has to continuously maintain the thoughtless state *nirvikalpa* through willpower, with constant awareness of this unity, by practicing yoga is a mantra. The limbs of Astanga Yoga—pranayama (breath control), yama (social discipline), niyama (individual discipline), dharana (concentration), dhyana (meditation), pratyahara (detachment), yoga (postures), and samadhi (mystical union with the divine)—are no longer used or required. All these are considered to be worthy and fruitful bodies of yoga at the beginning stages of the practices of yoga, or sadhna.

On the plane of Shambavopaya, there is nothing to do and nowhere to go. Yoga here can barely be called such; any yoga practiced here is essentially completed. There is actually no process, but by simply being on this plane, the Shakti Kundalini is uniting with Shiva at the crown of the head, affecting the ears and eyes. This meditative union of God is the form of hearing nada, or unstruck sounds, emitting through the Kundalini-filled Sushumna.

FOUR STAGES OF MAN'S LIFECYCLE IN VEDAS

1. Student life. When the student lives with his teacher and receives both religious and secular instructions. The youth is trained in self-control and acquires such virtues as chastity, truthfulness, and faith.
2. Married Life. In this stage mostly ritualistic sacrifices are practiced as explained in the Brahmanas.
3. Retired Life. This stage no longer requires adhering to ritualistic practices but needs to follow the Aranyakas, or the symbolic meditation.
4. Renunciation. In this fourth stage he is bound neither by work nor desire but is wholly dedicated to acquiring the knowledge of the Brahman. It is the spirit of self-abnegation in everything. However, it does not advocate renouncing normal life and retiring to the forest. It is rather the pivotal point around which the wheel of life should revolve. It enables one to carry the thought of God every moment of life.

The knowledge found here is not an end in itself but enables one to perform the actions that gain an end. The end gained always has limited results. However, through the institution of monasticism, a man may enter the life of renunciation at any stage. According to Vedic teachings, this monastic life is the highest stage a man may attain.

The Janana-Kanda is the second section of the Vedanta, the spiritual portion—the gist or the goal of the Vedas. The essence of the knowledge of the Vedas was called by the name Vedanta; it comprises the Upanishad. The word *Upanishad* translates as: Upa =near, ni =devotedly, shad=sitting. The highest wisdom can be learned by sitting devotedly at the feet of a teacher who himself possesses the knowledge and communicates the same to the world at large through secret channels. This means it imparts knowledge only to those who have attained purity of heart through following various self-discipline practices.

Speaking of the Upanishads, Schopenhauer comments: "In the whole world, there is no study so beneficial and so elevating as the Upanishads. It has been the solace of my life, it will be the solace of my life."[i] Schopenhauer, reflecting on the idea of will, has this to say: "All that exists for knowledge, and therefore the whole world, is only object in relation to subject, perception of a perceiver. This obviously is true of the past, future and present, of what is farthest off, as of what is near; for it is true of time and space themselves, in which alone these distinctions arise. All that belongs to the world is inevitable thus conditioned through the subject, and exist only for the subject. The Word is idea. The World is my will." The cause of creation was described as "that which existed at first become changed into will, and this will began to manifest itself as desire." The idea of will has been the cornerstone of Vedantic system.

THE CLASSIFICATION OF INDIAN PHILOSOPHY

There are twelve major schools of Indian philosophy. Some of these are grouped as follows:

A. **The Vedic: those who accept the authority of the Vedas are called Orthodox.**

B. **The Nonvedic: those who deny the authority of the Vedas are called Heterodox.**

A. The six Vedic (Orthodox) systems of philosophy

1) Nyaya
2) Vaisesika
3) Mimsa
4) Sankhya
5) Vedanta
6) Yoga

B. The three Nonvedic (Heterodox) systems of philosophy

1) Materialism
2) Jainism
3) Buddhism

A. THE SIX VEDIC (ORTHODOX) SCHOOLS OF PHILOSOPHY

All the six Indian philosophies consider the Upanishads as the final authority for all disputed doctrines of the Vedanta. All six schools assume that the Vedic philosophy must serve to release the embodied soul from an otherwise unending cycle of transmigration. Aside from these, each of the schools has a distinctive perspective. The following six philosophies are discussed briefly.

1. NYAYA

Nyaya means to investigate both physical and metaphysical subjects by and through analytic and logical methods. There are four sources of knowledge according to Nyaya: namely, perception, inference, analogy and authoritative testimony. The process of reasoning remarkably resembles the syllogistic analysis of Aristotle. Nyaya, the science of logical proofs, provides a well-founded system for the philosophical investigation of the object and the subject of human knowledge.

2. VAISESIKA

Vaisesika, the companion school of Nyaya, was established prior to it. The Vaisesika is more interested in cosmology. It claims all material objects are made of four kinds of atoms. Different combination of these atoms, namely earth, water, fire, and air, make different materials. In fact, there are nine substances, including the above-mentioned four material atoms. These include space, time, ether (akasha), mind, and self. It accepts a personal God. He created the world, but not out of nothing. A personal God set the atoms in motion.

3A. UTTARA MIMAMSA

Uttara Mimamsa is concerned with the attainment of knowledge. The most opposed factions have been compelled to take up the texts of Sage Vyasa and harmonize the text with their own philosophy. According to Vyasa, the powers of the God can be acquired by the liberated, but no one will acquire the power of creating, ruling, or dissolving the universe, since that power belongs to God alone.

3B. PURVA MIMAMSA

Purva Mimamsa (earlier investigation) was given the name to distinguish it from the Uttra (later) Mimamsa school. This school's most valuable contribution to Hinduism was its formulation of the rules of Vedic interpretations. Its adherents believed that reasoning must prove the revelation. Keeping this in mind, they laid great emphasis on dharma, which they understood as the performance of Vedic rituals. Sage Jaimini is regarded as the founder of Purva Mimamsa, which deals with the subject matter of rituals. The purification acts of rituals serves as preparation for the attainment of knowledge. It is the school of the ceremonial and of interpretation of sacrificial action.

4. SANKHYA PHILOSOPHY

The founder of the Sankhya philosophy is considered to be Rishi Kapila. The philosophy maintains two principles, namely that of

Purusa[1] and the second is the Prakriti. Sankhya philosophy divides the universe into twenty-five principles. The first eight comprise the material universe, termed *Prakriti*. One principle is the motive power of the universe, which is looked upon as soul or spirit and is termed *Purusha*. The remaining sixteen principles are the result of Purasha acting upon Prakriti, and they constitute the material universe, with all its movements of rotation, revolution, and gravitation. According to Sankhya, the Purusas are numerous and Prakriti is one. According to Sankhya, everything begins with Prakriti (matter), but this matter in itself is static. It is activated by the stimulus provided to it by the motive power from Purusha. The result of this is the manifested universe. This philosophy is very similar to nature. Everything is from nature, and nature is the cause of all manifestations, which we call thought, intellect, reason, love, taste, and matter. Nature consists of three elements called *Sattva, Rajas,* and *Tamas;* these are the materials out of which the whole universe has evolved. The first manifestation of Prakriti in the cosmos is what Sankhya calls *Mahat,* or intelligence. This intelligence itself is modified into what we call egoism, and this intelligence is the cause of all the powers in the body. It covers subconsciousness, consciousness, and superconsciousness; these are the three states in which knowledge exists. The chitt is the three-fold function of the mind, intelligence, and consciousness, which produces the force called *prana.* Pranas are the vital forces that manipulate the whole body, while they are manipulated by the mind or internal organs. Sankhya philosophy is basically the principle that one thing evolves out of another. According to this philosophy, the soul is infinite, the only thing not composed of matter. It is apparently bound by nature. The soul is identified with the nature. The soul has neither pleasure nor pain. According to Sankhya there is one eternal element; every other element is produced out of this one. It is called *akasha.* Along with this element there is the primal energy called prana. Akasha and prana combine and recombine to form

---

[1]   Purusha is neither intelligence nor will nor Mahat; it is the pure self.

elements. According to Sankhya, nature is omnipresent and contains the causes of everything that exists.[ii] In conclusion, there is no God as the Creator of the universe, according to Sankhya. Nature is sufficient by itself to account for everything.

5. VEDANTA

The fundamental principle of Vedanta is oneness, and that oneness is on the highest spiritual plane. According to Vedanta, there is one life which exists, one spirit, one truth, and one reality. Some people think that the Vedanta philosophy teaches that the world is an illusion. The Vedanta philosophy does not teach that the phenomenal world is such. What is regarded as illusion is the attribution of substantia and sentience to the phenomena, without recognizing the underlying unity, and that unity of being or existence. This, in Vedanta, is called by various names; it is called Brahman/absolute, which means a vast expanse—an infinite expanse. Plato called it, 'The Good'; Spinoza called it, the 'Substantia'; Spencer, 'the Unknown and Unknowable.' Kant called it the transcendental 'thing-in-itself.'[iii] Plato regards Good as the cause for existence for all things that exists and of knowledge to all minds that know them. Thus he suggests, the idea of Good is the ultimate cause or reason for the universe, and it must be the principle of unity in the consciousness of man. Of course, to draw an analogy between Plato and Vedanta we need to notice that in Plato's philosophy the idea of Good is more and more identified with God. Vedanta philosophy says, "If you wish to know the truth, do not seek for it outside, search within; there alone you will find the truth." Many religious philosophers think it is appalling to go beyond thought or to think there is any higher state of existence. According to Vedanta, there is a much higher state of existence, which is beyond thought and reasoning: when you step beyond thought and all reasoning, you have made the first step toward God. According to the Vedas, this is the beginning of life. The state beyond thought and reasoning is the highest state, upon which all the thoughts of humans stand.

6. YOGA SUTRAS OF MAHARISHI PATANJALI

Pathanjali, the founder of yoga philosophy, defines yoga as the elimination of the modifications of the mind; for him it is the separation between Purusha and Prakriti that brings liberation. From the analysis of the above definition and description of yoga, it is evident that the essential characteristic of yoga is brought about by two important processes or practices, which could bring about changes in the perception of the mind: constant practice and detachment. The two factors have also been described by Patanjali as a means for bringing calmness to the mind. The Yoga Sutras of Patanjali (300 BC) is treatise on methodological process for obtaining the goal laid down by Sage Kapila and adding something more to it. Kapila emphasizes knowledge, which involves only the mind; Patanjali's system involves both mind and body. In this respect the Purusha of Patanjali has to do two things simultaneously: one must acquire knowledge (Jananha) and one must also practice yoga in order to achieve excellence of both body and mind. By combining knowledge and yoga practices together, the individual will attain not only excellent health but will also be able to maintain a harmonious relationship between mind and the body. Thus it can be assumed that Patanjali's yoga provides a better and more thorough answer to our problems than what was perceived by the sage Kapila. Since Patanjali's system involves both knowing and doing, his method includes all those steps that are essential for obtaining the desired goal on both physical and mental levels.

Sage Patanjali, the writer of Yoga-Sutra, was, according to the ancient Indian mythology, an incarnation of Ananta, or Sesa, the thousand-headed leader of a serpent race. Ananta wanted to teach yoga on earth and is said to have fallen from Heaven onto the palm of a noble woman called Gonika. Ananta is often depicted as the couch on which Lord Vishnu takes repose. The numerous heads of the Lord of Serpents symbolize infinity or omnipresence. Sesa remains after the destruction of the cosmos. Patanjali wrote Yoga-Sutra at a time when there was ongoing debate on philosophy in India. The word *Sutra* means thread and indicates the threading together of short aphoristic statements. In Patanjali's work, the text of Yoga-Sutra consists of 195 sutras.

Patanjalis Yoga is not about the perfection of "technique," which may override the philosophical investigation, nor does yoga attempt to separate theory from the practice. But Patanjali's approach was to unite theory with practice, bridging between thinking and acting, metaphysics and ethics. Yoga-Sutra enumerates five afflictions (kleshas) and nine obstacles (vikshepas) as imperfections in the health of the body and in the state of mind. The philosophy of afflictions (kleshas) is the foundation of the system of yoga outlined by Patanjali. In its essential ideas it forms the substratum of all schools of yoga, though perhaps it has not been expounded as clearly and systematically as in the Samkhya and Yoga Darshanas.

Kleshas means pains, afflictions, or misery, but gradually it came to acquire the meaning of what causes pain, affliction, and misery. It is an analysis of the fundamental cause of human misery and suffering and the way in which this cause can be effectively removed. The Rishis who expounded this philosophy were great adepts who combined in themselves the qualifications of religious teacher, scientist, and philosopher. With their qualifications, they observed the phenomena of life not only with the help of their senses and minds, but in full conviction that the solution lay beyond even the intellect; they dived deeper into their own consciousness, tearing apart veil after veil until they discovered the ultimate cause of misery and suffering, which are inevitable. Avidya, or ignorance, is the root of kleshas. The self, which is eternally free and self-sufficient, is made to assume the limitation of Avidya by involving it with matter. Depriving the self of the knowledge or the awareness of its eternal and self-sufficient nature results in an inability to distinguish between the eternal, pure, blissful self and the non-eternal, impure, and painful. The word *eternal* means a state of consciousness that is above the limitations of time, while *pure* refers to the purity of consciousness as it is, unaffected and unmodified by matter, which is imposed upon it by the limitations of three Gunas, or modes. These impurities are in the nature of every human being. According to the Sankhya philosophy, nature is composed of three forces. In Sanskrit they are called Sattva, Rajas, and Tamas. All these are robbers, for they rob man of all his treasures and make him forget his true nature. In the physical world these three qualities may be called equilibrium, activity, and inertness. In all creation, animals, plants, and men, we find the manifestations of all the three forces. A yogi, also human, is affected by these three Gunas, but by his constant and disciplined study of himself and of the objects through his senses, he learns which thoughts, which words, and which actions are prompted by Tamas, which are Rajas, and which are Sattvaic. He who sees the three Gunas as the governing forces in all his actions, no doubt determined by the past karmas, transcends them by discrimination of the consciousness from those actions of the body and attains to the supreme consciousness. He sees the pure self in its essential nature, freed from birth, death, old age, and suffering, and experiences freedom. The text of Patanjali's Yoga-Sutra holds a specific place in the history of yogas. It is divided in four Padas, or chapters.

First Pada is called Samadi Pada: In this the goal of yoga is explained.

In second Sadhna Pada, some ways of practicing yoga to attain Samadhi are explained.

In the third Vibhuti Pada, the powers gained by Dharana, Dhyana, Samadhi (i.e., Samyam) are explained.

The fourth Kaivalya Pada is devoted to the explanation of Kaivalaya, or solace.

These texts are in the form of aphorisms but were commented upon by Sage Vyasa, Vachaspati, and Bhoja. The yoga-shastra was placed before the public in an extended form called *yoga-darsana*.

YOGA AND DIFFERENT SYSTEMS OF PHILOSOPHICAL THOUGHT

The philosophical thought of yoga found its roots in the Vedic Samhitas, Brahmanas, and Aranyakas and particularly in the Upanishads. All philosophical schools have been developed during the post-Vedic period. The number of schools is principally due to the attempts of various teachers to interpret the Upanishadic doctrines so as to form a consistent and intelligible system of thought. The schools of thought are called *Darsanas*. The word *Darsana'* indicates a vision of truth, a direct or immediate realization over and above ordinary perception. Thus these philosophical schools represent both theoretical and practical realization of the truth or goals aimed for. Both involve exercise and mind as primary faculties.

There are nine principal Darsanas, divided into two groups: orthodox and heterodox. All the Darsanas have a common goal of liberating man from Dhukhas, or suffering. Their philosophy is based on four common principles:

1. Human experiences are unsatisfactory and finally end in Dhukhas.
2. The cause of Dhukhas is avidya and avivek, or non-reasoning. A false relationship between the subject and the objects of experience, their attachments, and the feeling of "I" due to false knowledge is another cause of Dhukhka.
3. The third commonly accepted principle is an affirmation of the possibility of release from the condition of life known as Samsara, or past karmas. The life cycle is full of Dhukhas.
   The process of release consists of transforming perception, through which one comes to realize the true nature of reality and one's own identity. This state is called by different names: nirvana, liberation, solace, or freedom.
4. The fourth method of achieving the emancipated state involves physical austerities, as well as mental discipline and spirituality. And this technical process is called yoga.

DIFFERENT SCHOOLS OF YOGA

To classify the present systems of yoga, one finds differences of opinions among the scholars. The reason for that is that the yogas overlap and interpenetrate to such an extent that several classifications have validity. It is possible to use a system that incorporates several yogas directly and several others indirectly. Sri Aurobindo, a known scholar, attempted a synthesis to all the main yogas and expounded his approach eloquently in some of his writings. At this stage, the main yogas may be differentiated as follows:

1. Jnana Yoga—Union by knowledge
2. Bhakti Yoga—Union by love and devotion
3. Karma Yoga—Union by action and service
4. Mantra Yoga—Union by voice and sound
5. Yantra Yoga—Union by vision and form
6. Laya and Kundalini Yoga—Union by arousal of latent psychic nerve-force
7. Tantric Yoga—A general term for the physiological disciplines. Also union by harnessing sexual energy
8. Hatha Yoga—Union by bodily mastery
9. Raja Yoga—Union by mental mastery

Each of these types of yogas is suited to different temperaments or approaches to life. Though all the paths lead ultimately to the same destination—union with God, the absolute—the lessons of each of them need to be integrated if true wisdom is to be attained.

A student of yoga is not required to have any particular belief in a particular doctrine or dogma of any particular religion. Earnestness, sincerity, and faithful practice will bring good results.

1. JNANA YOGA

I shall tell you in full, of knowledge, speculative and practical, knowing which, nothing more here remains to be known. Bhagavad Gita

The yoga of knowledge or wisdom is the most difficult path, requiring tremendous strength of will and intellect. The word *Jnana* is derived from the Sanskrit word *Jna*, to know—in other words, knowledge. The ideal for the practitioner of this yoga is the realization of the absolute truth, and that is one common source for all subjective and objective phenomena in the universe. It teaches that all beliefs in the multiplicity of existence are unreal and illusory. Ignorance really means the undifferentiated consciousness that comes when we have no clear understanding or knowledge. And that kind of knowledge, taking the impermanent as permanent, is called ignorance. It can be removed by giving the right knowledge of the universal spirit. Jnana Yoga is also based on the monastic principles of Advaita, or the non-dualistic system of Vedanta. Its main purpose is to unify God and the individual soul and to show the oneness that exists between them on the higher spiritual plane. A Jnana yogi constantly practices discrimination and rises above all relativity and phenomenal worlds. He realizes the absolute, unchangeable, eternal truth in this life. Applying the philosophy of Vedanta, the Jnana yogi uses his mind to inquire into its own nature. We perceive the space inside and outside a glass as different, just as we see ourselves as separate from God. Janana Yoga leads the devotee to experience unity with God directly by breaking the glass, dissolving the veils of ignorance. Before practicing Janana Yoga, the aspirant needs to have integrated the lessons of the other yogic paths, for without selflessness, love of God, and strength of body and mind, the search for self-realization can become mere idle speculation. A true Janana yogi constantly tries to keep himself above all phenomenal conditions; he says within himself: I am neither mind, nor intellect, nor ego, nor senses, nor body. I am neither earth, nor water, nor air, nor fire, nor ether, but my true nature is absolute existence, knowledge, and bliss.

2. BHAKTI YOGA

Those who fix their mind on Me, worship Me, ever Steadfast and endowed with supreme Shraddha/faith, they in my opinion are best versed in Yoga. Bhagavad Gita

Bhakti means devotion, and Bhakti Yoga is the method of devotion resulting in true communion of the soul with the Supreme. Bhakti

Yoga is the path of devotion, which appeals particularly to those of an emotional nature. Bhakti Yoga is an embodiment of love. Through prayer, worship, and rituals, the devotee surrenders himself to God, channeling and transmitting his emotions into unconditional love or devotion. Chanting or singing the praises of God form a substantial part of Bhakti Yoga. A follower of Bhakti Yoga should feel God as closely related to his soul as he possibly can and regard him not only as the Lord of universe, but also as his father, mother, brother, sister, friend, or child. The yogi does not have the sense of I, me, and mine and makes room for thou and thee. The highest goal in Bhakti Yoga is infinite love for God. It regards man's natural power of love as a manifestation of the divine within and teaches him to purify that love until it becomes omnipotent. Devotion to God, to a higher superhuman power, has always stirred the heart of man. When the whole heart of a Bhakta, or love for God, flows like the unbroken current of a mighty river, he finds no attraction in the world, holds no other thought, cherishes no other desire, and sees no other object other than that of his own Deity. Every action of his body and mind is performed to please his beloved one. His motivational power is love alone, and by this he breaks the chain of selfishness, transcends the law of karma, and attains freedom.

3. KARMA YOGA

Man does not attain from action without entering action; nor does he reach perfection (without the discipline of knowledge) merely by ceasing to act. Bhagavad Gita

Karma Yoga is the method or science of attaining perfection through action or work. The Sanskrit word *karma* is derived from the root word *kri*, which means to act. So karma signifies action and refers to all actions, whether of mind or of body. Devotion, worship, meditation, and concentration are all "karma." Eating, talking, et cetera, is karma. Karma Yoga means the path of attainment to the union of lower self to the higher self through karma, or action. No cause can be isolated from its effects. It is the path chosen primarily by those of an outgoing nature. It purifies the heart by teaching you to act selflessly, without thought of gain or reward. By detaching yourself from the fruits of your actions and offering them to God, you learn to limit the ego. To achieve this, it is helpful to keep your mind focused by repeating a mantra while engaged in any activity. Bhagavad Gita says, "To work without seeking for the results of the work, which means disinterested work. It is our duty to work in the spirit of worship and not to ask for its results. Work as worship never binds a man in the chain of delusion; it rather emancipates him by the knowledge of the self."

By following this path of yoga, we can learn the secrets of how to utilize our daily actions to achieve the divine perfection that is inherent in us.

4. MANTRA YOGA

Mantras are words, phrases, or syllables that are chanted thoughtfully and with a great attention. Mantra Yoga involves chanting a word or phrase until the mind and desires are transcended. By the music of a mantra, the Sadhka's, or student's, mind gets immersed in the object of meditation. The rhythm and the meaning of a mantra combined together make the higher consciousness or a specific spiritual focus. By chanting a mantra, with its meaning as a thought, body, and consciousness, the yogi unites with the Supreme consciousness,

5. YANTRA YOGA

Yantra Yoga comes from Tibetan Buddhist tradition and is similar to Hatha Yoga. In Yantra Yoga the asanas, or postures, are important but not the main focus. Movement is more important. For example, in order to get into an asana, breathing and movement are linked and applied gradually. Hatha Yoga movement is also limited by time: a period to get into the position, a period to remain in that position, and a period to finish the position. Everything is related in Yantra Yoga. The overall movement is important, not only the asana.

6. LAYA YOGA AND KUNDILINI YOGA

In Laya Yoga, a student particularly needs a teacher who can locate the centers of energy, or the chakras. When these chakras are found, they function very much like doorways to different realms of higher consciousness.

Kundilini energy is one's dormant spiritual energy. In its dormant state it is visualized as a snake coiled up on the first chakra at the base of spine. The roused Kundilini energy moves upwards in the central Nadi, the Sushumana, passing through each of the lower chakras to reach the seventh, the Sahasrara chakra. This process is known in Kundalini Yoga as the piercing of the chakras and represents the merging of female with the male. Laya Yoga is also called Kundilini Yoga, because the raising of Kundalini energy to unite her with the supreme consciousness is the main objective, which is reached through deep meditation.

KUNDALINI AND ITS AWAKENING

Each chakra has a particular color, mantra, and symbol. In tantra and yoga, the chakras are symbolized by lotus flowers. There are different stages in spiritual life which represent different existences: ignorance, aspiration, and illumination. So does the lotus exist in three different levels: mud, water, and air. It sprouts in the mud (ignorance), grows up through the water (aspirations), and eventually reaches the air to the direct light of sun (illumination). In many of the practices of Kundalini Yoga we usually focus our awareness on the different chakras in the spinal cord, which creates a sensation, and that sensation passes through the Sushmana nadi and finally to the brain. Mooldhara chakra is the fundamental, or the root, where the evolution commences, and Sahasra is where the evolution is completed.

Since ancient times, the wise have realized that the mind can be expanded, and we do not need objects in order to experience. Tantra says that with the help of sense, one can have an experience based on and beyond the framework of time, space, and object. Tantrics and yogis have realized that in this physical body there exists a potential force called

Kundilini which is the consciousness of mankind. In Sanskrit, *kundal* means coil, and so kundalini is that which is coiled and comes from a deeper place, pit, or cavity. The word itself comes from Kunda. Kundalini resides in the Muladhara chakra. Usually with the awakening of kundalini the greater intelligence is aroused from its sleep, which affects the whole area of the human mind and behavior. A transformation takes place in life. By means of this transformation we speed up physical, mental, and spiritual evolution. Once the great Shakti awakens, man is no longer a gross physical body with a lower mind; we become conscious of the world, which is full of willpower, thought, knowledge, and action. Values in life also change, relationships improve, and the higher qualities of compassion and contentment are also gained. Before commencing with Kundalini Yoga we must try to find out where we should start; the method is to concentrate on the Muladhara chakra and then Swadhisthana, and so on. By doing this we can discover the point of evolution of our thought. The purpose is to awaken all the chakras and their related other small chakras. A yogi practicing yoga as a mantra in the subtle energetic realm is practicing in the deepest stillness and with inner silence if possible. At this Shambavopaya plane, Shakti Kundalini is uniting with Shiva at the crown of the head. Therefore the objects of meditative union of Shiva and Shakti take a form inner hearing of Nada, the un-struck sounds emitted through the Kundalini-filled Sushumna.

7. TANTRIC YOGA

The word *tantra* means a rule, a teaching, or technical system. Its root meaning is to control, or harness; therefore, it teaches us not to suppress the forces of reality but to control and harness them. One of the characteristic of the tantric approach, which is Shyesavism, exemplifies honoring the natural unfolding of life. In Shiva Tantra, a yogi will use natural pleasures—music, food, and sexuality—as doorways to divinity. Kashmiri Shavism has four schools: Kula, Krama, Spadina, and Pratyabhijna. Kula and Krama are the older Tantric schools. In the twentieth century a great yogi and a scholar, Swami Lakshman ju, a

Brahmin, learned the ancient texts of Shavism in Sanskrit and was not content with its intellectual knowledge only. As the texts and teachings permeated him, they detonated an inner explosion. Swami Lakshman ju of Srinagar was transformed, so much so that those who studied with him later experienced him as an enlightened master.

Tantra is an ancient philosophy interpreted as an act of sexuality, though the philosophy is to treat our partner as a divine and spiritual being. It is a path to spiritual enlightenment, but unfortunately in some societies, a version has been secularized to help couples bond.

8. HATHA YOGA

The word *Hatha* derives from two roots: *ha* means sun and *tha* means moon. The flow of breath in the right nostril is called the sun breath and the flow of breath in the left nostril is the moon breath. Central to all Hatha Yoga disciplines is the regulation of breath, harmonizing of its positive (sun) and negative (moon), or male and female, currents. Another meaning of Hatha is forced, but the term Forced Yoga would not do justice to the poised and gentle nature of most yogic controls. In Hatha Yoga we mainly deal with yoga asanas, kriyas (cleansing processes), mudras, pranayamas (regulation of breath), and meditation. Hatha Yoga may be viewed as a hygiene that takes into account the purification of the total organism.

Raja Yoga begins where Hatha Yoga, if properly followed, ends. It would therefore be unwise to consider Hatha Yoga as nothing more than a dangerous gymnastic feat, for a moderate exercise of it has been found by experience to be both conductive to health and longevity. It brings the power to prevent or remove diseases, physical or mental, for its practice regulates the action of the heart and the lungs and the circulation of blood. It even bestows the gift of putting off death indefinitely, although this privilege is seldom exercised by the true yogi, who knows the consequences of interfering with the laws of nature.

Raja and Hatha Yoga are the necessary counterparts of each other, the limbs, as it were, of the same body. Either of them cannot be successfully followed to the exclusion of the other, nor their benefits be secured without the direction of a learned teacher; no one can be a perfect yogi without knowledge of the practices of both.

Hatha Yoga identifies the six destroyers of yoga practice:

1. Overeating
2. Overexertion
3. Useless talk
4. Undisciplined conduct
5. Bad company
6. Restless inconstancy

To overcome the hurdles, Patanjali offers this four-fold remedy:

1. Friendly attitude toward all
2. Compassion with devoted action
3. Appreciation of good work done by others
4. Removal of feeling superior to others

9. RAJA YOGA

For the Sage who wishes to ascend to Dhyana Yoga, action is said to be the means, when he has ascended to Dhyana yoga, inaction alone is said to be the means. Bhagavad Gita

Raja means the king; it is the king of all the yogas. This yoga teaches us how to concentrate our minds on one chosen object and how to develop the power of meditation. Its aim is to remove all mental obstructions, gain a perfectly controlled healthy mind, strengthen the willpower, and to lead the seeker after truth through the path of concentration and meditation to the ultimate goal. Raja Yoga is the science of physical and mental control. It offers a comprehensive method for controlling the waves of thought by turning our mental and physical energy into spiritual energy.

Raja Yoga is closely associated with the systematization of yoga techniques by Patanjali in his Yoga-Sutra. He lists asanas and pranayama among his "eight limbs" of yoga, and such classic texts as the Hatha Yoga Pradipika, the Gheranda Samhita, and the Shiva Samhita follow Patanjali in seeing Hatha Yoga practices as providing a physiological hygiene that prepares the body for effective mental control. According to this view, Raja Yoga includes Hatha Yoga within its system. Hatha Yoga works upon the body, purifying and perfecting it, and through the body upon the mind. Raja Yoga works upon the mind, refining it and perfecting it, and through the mind upon the body. The highest authority on Raja Yoga is the ancient Sage Patanjali (this yoga is based on Sankhya philosophy). Patanjali says that God can be the subject of concentration and meditation. Perfection in Raja Yoga means the attainment of that state of consciousness in which there is no bondage, no limitation, no imperfection of any sort. Patanjali considers that Raja Yoga is composed of eight limbs, or steps, called Astanga Yoga. These are the progressive series of steps and disciplines that purify the body and the mind and ultimately lead yogin to enlightenment.

THE STEPS OF ASTANGA YOGA

1. Yamas (abstinence)
2. Niyamas (observances)
3. Asanas (postures)
4. Pranayama (breath control)
5. Pratyahara (Sense withdrawal)
6. Dharana (concentration)
7. Dhyana (contemplation)
8. Samadhi (self-realization)

SOCIAL DISCIPLINE: YAMAS

Ahimsa (nonviolence)
Astheya (non-stealing)

Satya (truthfulness)
Brahmacharya (continence)
Apargraha (non-coveting)

AHIMSA (NONVIOLENCE)

To not cause injury to any living being through thought, word, or deed. Our attitude must always be nonviolent. In other words, love of the entire creation is Ahimsa. We should practice the golden rule: do unto others as you wish others to do unto you.

ASTHEYA (NON-STEALING)

To not steal anything and not envy others' wealth or possessions. Do not think or ask for what you should not have. Do not claim a thing that is not yours. Do not keep with you more than your minimum needs.

SATYA (TRUTHFULNESS)

Satya is saying what one sees with one's own eyes, hears with one's own ears, and understands through one's own brain. It means that truthfulness should not only be external but internal also.

BRAHMACHARYA (CONTINENCE)

A Brahmacharya is one who moves in Brahman, or God, or lives in Brahman, or God, whose mind is fixed on Brahman, the absolute, the supreme being, and who preserves continence. To keep one's sense organs, including the organs of procreation, under control and not to be tempted by lustful enjoyments through thought, word, and deed.

APARIGRAHA (NON-COVETING)

Accept what you have and do not ask for more. In Asteya, one gives up stealing but accepts charity. But in Aparigraha, chastity is not accepted. We should not exaggerate or multiply our needs, but learn to be satisfied with our basic requirements.

INDIVIDUAL DISCIPLINE: NIYAMAS

Saucha (purity, cleanliness)
Santosha (contentment)
Tapas (discipline or self-control)
Swadhaya (study of scriptures)
Isvara Pranidhana (devotion to Lord)

SAUCHA (PURITY, CLEANLINESS)

Saucha implies purity, internal and external. Purity of mind is specially emphasized. The body can be kept clean by pure Sattavic food, and there are six types of yogic purifications. Mind's purity is achieved through giving up attachments, jealousy, and other ideas.

SANTOSHA (CONTENTMENT)

One should be content with whatever is required while truthfully doing one's duty or whatever is received through the grace of God. We must be detached from pleasure and pain and so preserve a balance in our life.

TAPAS (SELF-CONTROL)

Tapas is a challenge to those who seek the higher life. Tapas literally means heat, an inner fire or energy that enables us to control body and mind. This power is created by ascetic practices, such as fasting, silence, and self-discipline.

SWADHAYA (STUDY OF SCRIPTURES)

It is the study of spiritual books like Upanishads, Gita, Bible, Qur'an, et cetera, to gain the real knowledge and spending time in the company of holy men and sages, exchanging ideas with them.

ISWARA PRANIDHANA (DEVOTION TO LORD)

It is the complete surrender of self to God in words, deeds, and thought. It implies worshiping God, chanting of his name, hearing about him, and thinking of him as all-pervasive, omnipresent, and omniscient. The god to whom Patanjali refers is more specifically a god of yogins. God's role in yoga is a teacher or master who can bring Samadhi to the yogin and who takes him as an object of his concentration. No doubt there are yogins who go beyond the stages of Samadhi without any guidance but by their willpower—perhaps that is the supreme yoga. This being a supreme form of devotion, a yogin at that time is in a plane of complete surrender of his own willpower to the Absolute/God.

ASANAS (POSTURES)

Any steady and comfortable pose is asana. Steady pose gives concentration of mind. By asana, Patanjali Maharishi means the seat or posture for meditation and says that a posture should be steady and pleasant. In order to attain a steady and pleasant posture, there are asanas that predispose the body for meditative posture. In Raja Yoga, asanas are steady meditative postures, whereas in Hatha Yoga, the whole organism receives attention from a wide range of postures, improving suppleness and flexibility.

PRANAYAMA (BREATH CONTROL)

Life begins with the first breath and terminates with the cessation of breath. Controlling the motion of inhalation and exhalation is called pranayama. Pranayama is the restraint of prana, or vital energy, by restraint of breath. Prana is controlled. This should not be taken literally. Suspension of breathing is a part of pranayama; it prepares the mind for meditation. It calms the mind-stuff, or chitta. Pranayama indicates that it is restraint of prana, the life force. Negative and positive pranic currents in the body are equalized and channeled in the Hatha Yoga practices. Pranayama in combination with the preceding stages prepares the mind for concentration, contemplation, and self-realization, which are the internal meditative techniques whereby the light of Purusha is uncovered. But first there is the initial process of turning inward, called pratyahara.

PRATYAHARA (SENSE WITHDRAWAL)

Sense withdrawal is, as it were, the sensors imitating the thinking principle by withdrawing themselves from their objects. Vivekananda describes it as: "when the senses have withdrawn from their objects and transmitted themselves into the modes of consciousness, this is called the withdrawal."

DHARANA (CONCENTRATION)

It is fixing the mind on an external object or an internal point. It is the retention or holding together of the collected consciousness for some time. Through dharana you can send the flow of blood to any part of your body. You can control the circulation of blood. With the help of concentration, you can send your whole mind to God, the divine, and thereby withdraw yourself from material body.

SAMADHI (PURE CONSCIOUSNESS)

Samadhi means a state of pure consciousness. It is the union of God or the absolute. The state of samadhi is beyond description. There is no means or language to give expression to it. In samadhi, the meditator looses his individuality and becomes identical with the absolute; the meditator and the meditated become one. Just as the river joins the ocean, the individual soul joins the Supreme soul, the ocean of absolute consciousness. In the state of samadhi, the aspirant is not conscious of any external or internal objects. There is no thinking, hearing, smelling, or seeing.

DHYANA (MEDITATION)

Meditation follows concentration, and concentration merges in meditation. Meditation, concentration, and samadhi are internal sadhanas. When you practice all three together, it is called *samyama*.

Meditation is freeing the mind from all thoughts of sense objects. During meditation, the mind dwells on the object alone. It is the constant remembrance of the object of meditation flowing like an unbroken stream of oil poured out from one vessel to the other. Dhayana is more important for spiritual realization, and it is essential for attaining the last step of Raja Yoga. The objective of meditation is to understand the real meaning and to realize it—to not merely know it intellectually, but to feel it and to be one with the ideal.

Meditation is a fully conscious process, an exercise of will. It also means concentration on a spiritual idea, thought, or a mantra, which involves the capability of rising above worldly, day-to-day matters. Meditation is the practice that engages constant observation of the mind. We try to focus the mind on one point of meditation in order to perceive only that object by stopping the thought waves in our mind. In major cases they are the desires. By this practice we come to understand our true nature and thereby discover the wisdom and tranquility that lie within us. While focusing on a chosen object of meditation, with the help of discrimination of thought, elimination of desires is linked to the worldly objects. A circle of thoughts or waves is made around our mind.

Practice, or abhyasa, plays a significant role; it can reduce the radius of the circle of thought waves to only one thought. According to the ancient Vedas, dharana, or concentration, is fixing the mind on one thought or one image for twelve seconds. Meditation, or dhyana, is equal to twelve dharanas, which is about two and a half minutes. Samadhi is twelve dhyanas—just under half an hour.

It is important to meditate on some energy centers, or chakras, especially the heart chakra anahata, or ajna, the third eye chakra. By practicing meditation, or dhyana, in this manner, our desires are soon eliminated, and our thoughts become merged with the divine or the object of our meditation. Thus, there is no subject and object relationship. We experience the infinite, the absolute unending, without any beginning or any end. We transcend our physical body and the world surrounding us. We see that our consciousness merges with the pure consciousness. Though that plane of existence may be yet far away, by following the path of a yoga with the strict austerities of Yamas and Niyamas, we can indeed reach that plane.

In order to meditate on the divine, we need to purify our mind. The centers of energy, or chakras, must be activated in order for a yogi to dwell on the higher planes of thoughts. Rhythmic breathing is very helpful. Mind and breath are always related and interact with each other. Pranayama is the most important discipline a student should constantly practice, which culminates into controlling thought, word, and body.

YOGIC PHYSIOLOGY OF BODY

According to the yogic physiology, the human body is divided in three categories: namely, the physical, subtle or astral, and casual body.

THREE TYPES OF BODIES

The physical body can be taken care by eating healthy and appropriate food. We also can control our physical body by regular practice of yoga and pranayama. By these practices we can attain a healthy state of our physical body.

The astral or subtle body is related to our mind and the energy chakras. The astral or subtle body can be controlled by paranayama and meditation on a regular basis.

The casual body is the finest body. It contains the consciousness itself and its connection to pure consciousness, or the absolute. This consciousness can be attained by the regular practice of meditation leading toward the ultimate state of emancipation.

FIVE COVERINGS (SHEATHS) OF THE BODY

According to the Yog-shaastra, all the three bodies mentioned above are covered with five layers, or sheaths, of energy. Each of these layers contains different aspects of the body. The knowledge of Yog-shaastras helps us to understand what consciousness is and how our bodies move from physical to subtle and casual body. By understanding these five layers of energy we can come nearer to our true identity. The knowledge of these energy layers and the body itself as an energy system helps us to become aware of our body as a manifestation of our spirit; thereby we can read our physical body like a scripture. The energies inside the universe vibrate with certain frequencies; these energies contain information about both the internal and external experiences of each one of us. This is only possible because these energies are in communication with everything around us, which creates a relationship with the people surrounding us, and also the energies beyond our planet.

As per the philosophy of yoga, there are seven energy chakras in a human body, the stages to higher spiritual consciousness. These seven mystical numbers define how we control and direct these energies to realize our own ethical and moral values, leading to a right relationship to ourselves, to others, to life, and to the Divine. The energy of this truth also vibrates within our biological constitution. This in turn directs us to the proper use of our energies. The path leading to this is through the practice of yoga, meditation, pranayama, and asanas. This makes us biologically Divine, and we achieve the final state of evolution.

PHYSICAL SHEATH: ANNAMAYA KOSHA (PHYSICAL BODY)

Our body is made up of five elements, or panciamaha-bhutas. Due to the presence of ego, the body undergoes transformations: birth, growth, diseases, old age, decay, and death and manifests qualities like fat or thin, white or black, young or old, healthy or sick, attractive or unattractive. We feel separate from the self.

It is our responsibility to take care of this sheath and redefine our relationship with our body through the regular practice of yoga asanas and proper Ayurvedic diet. There are some recommended asanas to establish control of our physical body.

VITAL SHEATH: PRANAMAYA KOSHA (ASTRAL BODY)

This is the next layer, where movement of our pranic forces directs our physical and mental activities. Vital energy is responsible for our physiological functions and life. Due to the presence of the ego, our body functions become imbalanced. To restore the balance, some yogic methods of purification are recommended.

MIND SHEATH: MANOMAYA KOSHA (ASTRAL BODY—LOWER MIND)

This sheath is the energy of actions; it is composed of two qualities: the mind and the intellect. Those individuals who reside in this layer are subject to experiencing pain, pleasure, longings, doubts, fear, and many tides of emotion. When the mind is cheerful, we are happy; when it is gloomy, we are depressed. This is because we bestow all the powers to the mind and make it our master. This sheath, the monomaya kosha, can be controlled by breath control and by meditation with total devotion.

INTELLECT SHEATH: VIJNANMAYA KOSHA (ASTRAL BODY—HIGHER MIND)

It is the sheath of the intellect and intuitive knowledge, which gives us reasoning capabilities and helps to differentiate between virtues and vice, good and bad, right and wrong.

The practice of meditation, regular self-study, and enrichment of knowledge can lead to the experiences of this layer. Ultimately we can discover that the self is different from the body.

BLISS SHEATH: ANANDAMAYA KOSHA (CASUAL BODY)

When we have transcended the above four layers, we begin to experience a sense of joy that is independent of any sensory input or past experiences or impressions. This kosha contains the essence of an individual soul's experiences of countless lifetimes and stages of spiritual evolution. A yogi who resides in this sheath of bliss experiences absolute peace, joy, and love.

TYPE OF YOGA ACCORDING TO THE NEEDS OF THE BODY

1. Persons with gross tendencies, animal instincts, interested only in body-building processes and developing the Anna-maya take recourse with Hatha Yoga.
2. Persons afflicted with wind or gastric troubles take recourse with the help of Pran Yoga.
3. Persons with mental impurity, ignorance, and modulations of the mind can take recourse with Raja Yoga.
4. Persons with a strong intellectual bent of mind can take the path of Jnana or Yoga of knowledge.
5. Those who are anxious to escape from the world and seek bliss for its own sake can follow the path of Anand Yoga, or Sehaj Yoga, or yoga of tree.

YOGA AND ITS SECRETS

Yoga is neither a religion nor a mysticism. It is the wisdom of life and experience. Yoga is the intelligent and self-conscious effort of man toward achieving universal existence. Yoga is a complete life; it is a timeless, a pragmatic science, evolved over thousands of years, dealing with the physical, moral, mental, and spiritual well-being of man as a whole. Yoga is for all human beings and is universal. The main objective of yoga is to teach mankind the different methods of attaining the knowledge of the self and the daily practices for self-control. The practice of self-control would be a great blessing to all mankind for leading a healthier and meaningful life. Yoga brings physical and mental efficiency, balance, and peace of mind. It confers eternal bliss, perfection, perennial joy, and everlasting peace. According to Bhagavad Gita: "It is the union of individual soul with the universal spirit and state of equipoise and skill in action."

Yoga was originally used to designate a union, or a connection between verses and words. Similarly various texts go by names of sutras. Brahmans and Aranyakas used the word yoga in the sense of conjunction or connection. With the growth of philosophical ideas during the Rig Veda period, people used to practice austerities. All these practices indicate the control of senses and, by their implications, also the control of mind. The root of *Yuj* is supposed to mean at least two things: to control (yuj-samyamad) and to contemplate (yuj-samadhau). Thus the word *yoga* is derived separately from two different roots, namely *yugir* and *yuj*, the former indicating a non-technical meaning used in ancient Vedic period and the latter with the quite technical meaning of controlling the senses and mind. The control of passion and anger comes when the mind does not seek pleasure from external objects but learns by experience that pleasure that can be derived through the senses is very transient; it lasts only temporarily, and its true source is not the object itself but depends mostly upon the mental and physical conditions of the pleasure seeker. The more objects of desire are gratified, the more desire will increase. If a person were to possess all the objects upon this earth, still man's greed would not end; he would seek something more. Perfect self-control, where no desires or passions of any kind disturb the peace and tranquility of man—such a state can be acquired by removing the bubbles of desire before they take the form of wave passions; that is, by attacking them while they are in their weak state. This can be done through the right type of discrimination of the nature of desires. Another way of obtaining self-control is through concentration and meditation.

RELEVANCE OF YOGA IN DAY-TO-DAY LIFE

In this modern age, the search for peace has interested masses of people in the benefits of meditation, pranayama, and yoga asanas. In the last few decades yoga has helped millions of people to improve their self-concept. Through yoga, man realizes that a man is not only the mind but also body and thought; therefore happiness is not experienced by mind alone. But mind and body alone are not adequate to experience happiness. This is because man, in addition to mind and body, also consists of emotions and desires. Man is sometimes beyond mind and psyche. Therefore yoga has been designed in such a way that it can complete the process of evolution of personality in every possible direction.

Although it seems like an abstract subject to many, yoga has assumed newer dimensions and greater relevance in today's jet-set world, because unlike a physical routine or an aerobic exercise, the aim of yoga is Sampurna Arogya, or total health. The practices of yoga are designed to guide a novice systematically and progressively through the various stages for attaining the goal of a healthy and robust life. Yoga is the perfect method to fight both congenital as well as acquired diseases, for which even modern allopathic medicines have only limited cures.

YOGA PRACTICES/SADHNA

All mantras in Vedas support a special type of yoga whose essence is the inner journey, or Yajna. A journey or kind of a sacrifice, it is the outer symbol of an inner work. It is an interchange between God and a human, man giving what he has and God in return giving power and light and winning victory in battle against the darkness and falsehoods on his behalf. Yajna, or the journey, also refers to the journey from the world of matter to the word of light and wisdom. A man who does Yajna reaches different states of consciousness, gets priceless experiences, and brings them back to the ordinary living conditions, thus making the human life divine. It is climbing from one degree of perfection to another; it is a battle, because there are some powers that hinder our journey toward perfection. These powers are called as dasyus, or destroyers, like Vrtra and Vala—demons, or simply the negative energies. People who do not recognize the principle of Yajna come under their influence; Yajna foster in them qualities like jealousy, greed, lust, and so on. Yajna is also connected with a mantra to reach the Absolute. We have to invoke the cosmic power in the inner sacrifice by a voice potent with the power of a mantra. To them we offer whatever is ours; in return we receive all that is given, thus reaching our goal. The mystic path to reach the Absolute is described as:

Anveshtavyo Brhaddivas Pantha

Which means:

The path is far wider and broader for the one who searches for the truth. In other words, supreme consciousness, which is beyond the truth (or satyam), truth of being; a path leading to felicity and immorality; it is in its right (rtam) activity both of mind and body. It is vast (brhat), infinite. It is beyond the three realms of the phenomenal existence: the earth, mid-region, and the sky.

These three realms constitute the lower half of reality. Beyond this is the upper half, where Surya sun is not only an image, but reigns and shines brilliantly; thus is the only reality (ekam sat). The greatest name man ever gave to God is Truth; through truth everything is attained. In truth everything is established.

The yoga practices of pranayama and meditation, and asanas are virtuous and give rise to experiences that are pleasant. In nature, the effect is always related to the cause and corresponds exactly to the cause that has set in motion. Since karma is a natural law, we can predict the karmic results of our actions and thoughts by imagining their consequences.

It may be pointed out at this time that Sage Patanjali has not attempted to give us a general idea concerning the Yoga-Sutra, but his objective is merely directed to the underlying cause of human suffering, so that we may be able to appreciate the means adopted in the yogic disciplines for its effective removal. The path does not matter; it is the attainment of the goal that is important.

The path lies in the world of phenomena, and a yogi can cut short the process of its unfolding and attain perfection. He can step out of the broad road and take a shortcut, though it is difficult. But following the path of yoga stops the generation of new personal karmas.

USEFUL RULES FOR YOGA PRACTICES

1. Time
    Asanas can be performed at any time, but morning is the best, as mind remains calm.

2. Place
    A pure, calm, and secluded place is best place for asanas. The room should be well ventilated.

3. Clothes
    Clothes should be loose and comfortable. Cotton is recommended.

4. Food
    Yoga should be practiced on an empty stomach.
    Food can be taken ten to fifteen minutes after completion of yoga practices

5. Stretching
    Do not overstretch, but start with simple asanas.

6. Pain
    In case of pain and discomfort, discontinue the practice.

7. Fasting
    A fast every week or once a fortnight gives the digestive system a much needed rest. At the same time it gives the body a chance to cleanse itself of accumulated toxins.

YOGA ASANAS WITH ANIMAL NAMES

In order to acquire some of the skills necessary for survival, the Rishis and yogis of yore closely studied animals and their attributes and behaviors. They practiced, perfected, and fully developed them in a form that today is known as yoga asanas. We find many of the asanas are named after the animals.

In ancient India, animals were obscured in nature and were noted for their particular abilities and accomplishments. To imitate these qualities was considered a high sign of spiritual wisdom. That is why so many yoga poses are named after animals and plants.

Some of the names of yoga asanas written in Sanskrit are as follows:

- Bakasana—Crow pose
- Bhekasana—Frog pose
- Bhujangasana—Cobra pose
- Gomukhasana—Cow face pose
- Kapotasana—Pigeon pose
- Kukkutasana—Cock pose
- Kurmasana—Tortoise pose
- Matsyasana—Fish pose
- Mayurasana—Peacock pose
- Nakrasana—Crocodile pose
- Adho Mukha Svanasana—Downward-facing dog pose
- Sinhasana—Lion pose
- Vatayanasana—Horse pose
- Vrschikasana—Scorpion pose
- Ushtrasana—Camel pose
- Garudasana—Eagle Pose
- Bidalasana—Cat pose

These poses, or asanas, are linked to their animal names and are inspired by the actions or anatomy of the animals after which they were named.

YOGA IS A MANTRA

SCIENCE OF THE INTERNAL REALM SINCE CREATION

"It is just a reminder to return home, and the practice of Kashmiri Yoga is to return home to the heart of what is natural."

Lalit Kilam

YOGA ASANAS IN DAY-TO-DAY LIFE

May Almighty confer health, strength and success on all those who take to the practice of yoga. Saluting the sun is a gesture of gratefulness to the sun's brightening, warming, and energizing nature and its effect s on our lives. Sun Salutations are done to the rising sun with folded hands, facing the east. We salute the Sun God for success in the performance of different asanas and in our life.

SUN SALUTATIONS
"Surya Namaskara"

Surya means Sun, and Namaskara refers to greetings or prayers. Surya Namaskara is a known mode of worship of Surya and is done at the rising of the sun. Surya Namaskara is a graceful sequence of twelve positions performed as a continuous flow of water. We should be practicing it facing the morning sun, bathing our whole body in the life-giving rays of the sun, the giver of life, light, joy, and warmth to the whole world.

Surya Namaskara is done after the utterance of *Om* with the appropriate mantra, along with the corresponding name of the sun God. The sun being the most unrestrained and life-giving force for the planet, it forms the visible representation of the invisible Almighty.

There are twelve sacred mantras uttered, and for each mantra one complete namaskara is done. There are twelve mantras for Surya Namaskar:

1. Om mitraya namah
2. Om ravaye namah
3. Om suryaya namah
4. Om bhanave namah
5. Om khagaya namah
6. Om pushne namah
7. Om hiranyagarbhaya namah
8. Om marichaya namah
9. Om adityaya namah
10. Om savitre namah
11. Om arkaya namah
12. Om bhaskaraya namah

The Sun Salutation, or Surya Namaskara, limbers up the whole body in preparation for the asanas. It is a graceful sequence of twelve positions performed as one continuous exercise. Each position counteracts the one before, stretching the body in a different way and alternately expanding and contracting the chest to regulate the breathing.

There are altogether eighty-four asanas, which purify the body, thoughts, and words and also have curative effects. Through the practice of different asanas, different afflictions vanish, and the gates of spirit of wisdom are opened.

SUN SALUTATIONS
"Surya Namaskara"

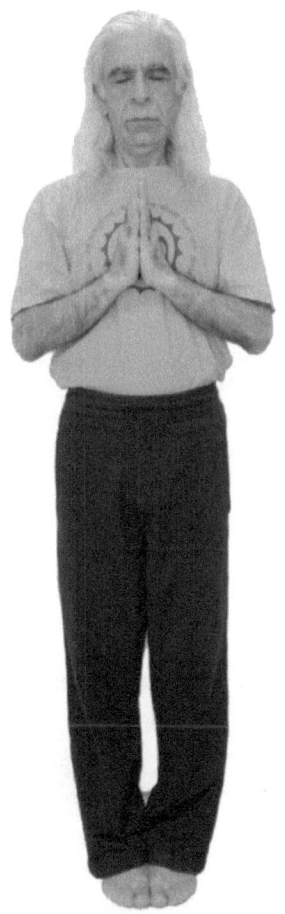

Position 1

Step 1 Process
- Stand with feet together and hands folded in front of the chest

"Surya Namaskara"

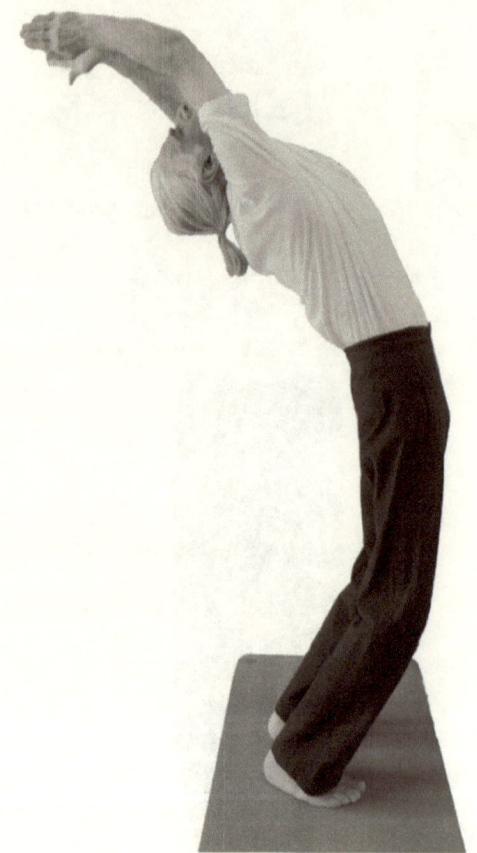

Position 2

Step 2 Process
- Raise hands and bend backward

"Surya Namaskara"

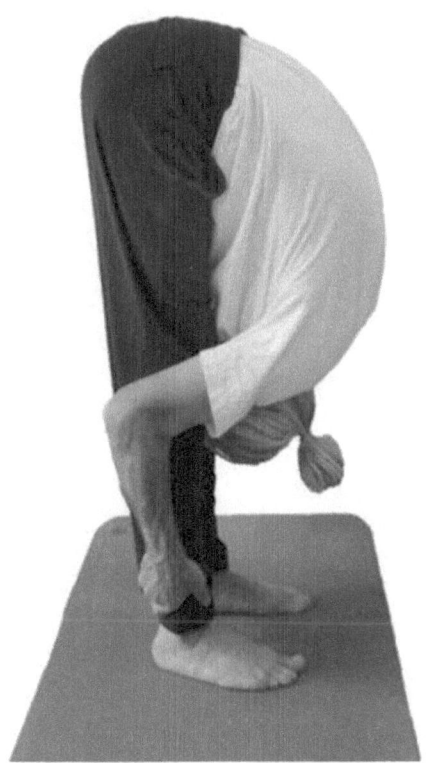

Position 3

Step 3 Process
- Bend forward and place hands on the ankles
- You may bend the knees if necessary in the beginning

"Surya Namaskara"

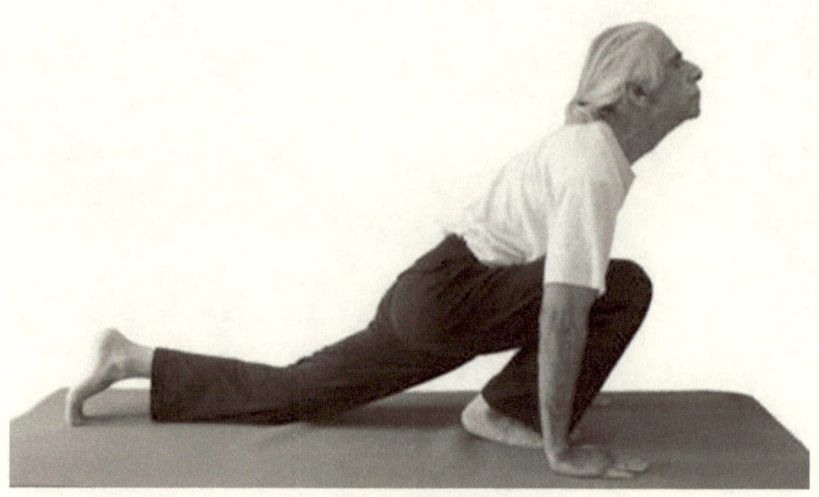

Position 4

Step 4 Process
- Stretch the left leg back while bending the right knee and lowering the torso
- Stretch the neck backward

"Surya Namaskara"

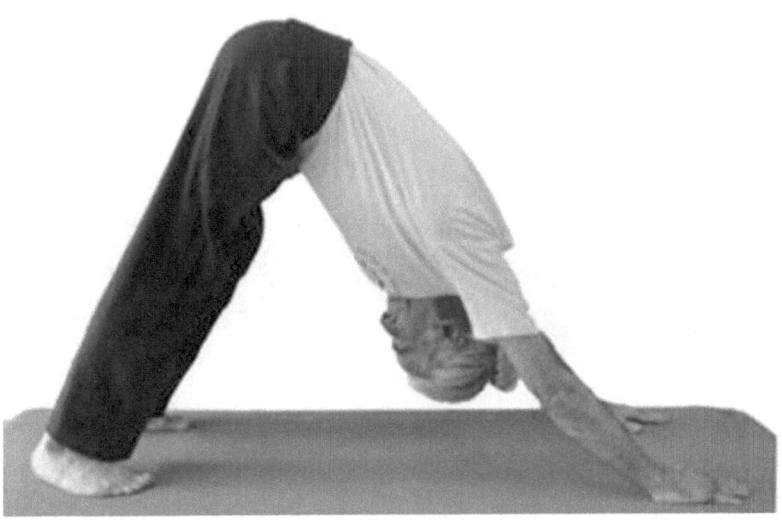

Position 5

Step 5 Process
*   Lifting the hips, move the right foot back to join the left foot
*   Lower your head
*   The body assumes a triangular position

"Surya namaskara"

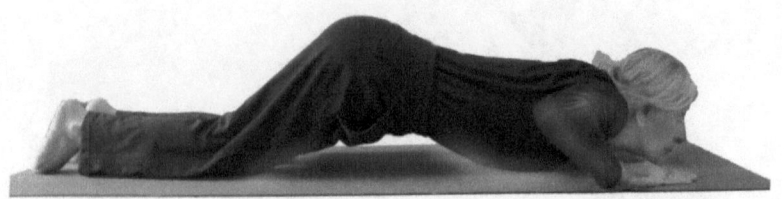

Position 6

Step 6 Process
- Lower the body to the floor
- Let the chin, chest, and knees rest on the floor
- Lift the hips and waist, bend the neck, and look at the navel

"Surya Namaskara"

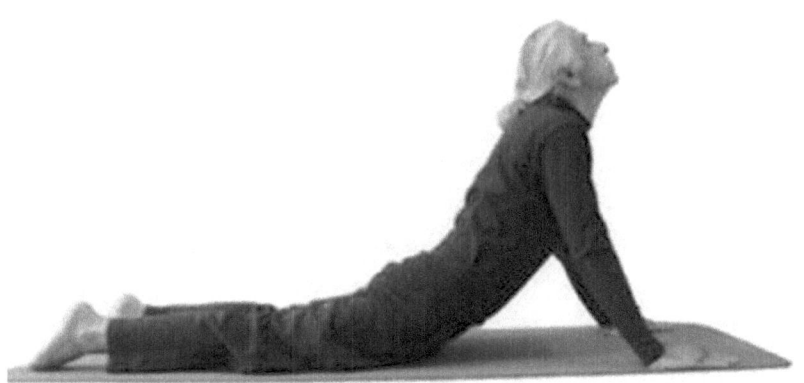

Position 7

Step 7 Process
- Drop the stomach
- Lift the head and raise the upper body
- The abdomen should remain on the floor
- Repeat position 5 which becomes position 8. Similarly repeat position 4; 3; 2; and 1 which become position 9; 10; 11; and 12

BENEFITS OF SURYA NAMASKARA

Each position of Surya Namaskara complements the one before, stretching the body in different ways and alternately expanding and contracting the chest to regulate the breathing. It provides the foundation for all culture of body, mind, and spirit. It makes the stomach, intestines, pancreas, and heart healthy. It also makes the spinal cord and the waist flexible and regulates the blood circulation in the entire body. It is also useful for diabetes. Surya Namaskara gives complete health to the body. All the activities of Surya Namaskara are synchronized with breathing. And each asana should be done with full awareness. All the mantras associated with the twelve positions of Surya Namaskara must be chanted, audibly or inaudibly. Chanting these mantras with single-minded devotion has an infinite effect on the personality of a student.

PADMASANA
"Lotus Pose"

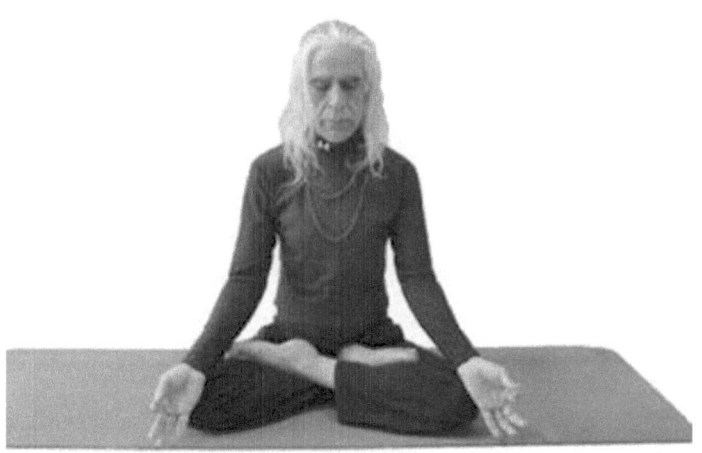

In Sanskrit, '*padma*' means lotus. This posture is called "Padmasana 'because the arrangement of the legs, hands, and feet resembles a lotus. The lotus flower is the symbol of purity and balance. It is the destroyer of all diseases. It is the most relaxing pose. The Kundalini Divine cosmic energy in the body is roused by this posture. Padmasana is a meditative posture.

BENEFITS OF PADMASANA

Padmasana maintains a balanced flow of energy throughout the body. This posture strengthens the thighs and calves and provides elasticity to the muscles. It helps to cure many heart and lung diseases. It helps to cure rheumatism of the legs. It also helps to reduce excess fat in the abdomen, buttocks, and thighs.

SIDDHASANA
"The posture of an adept"

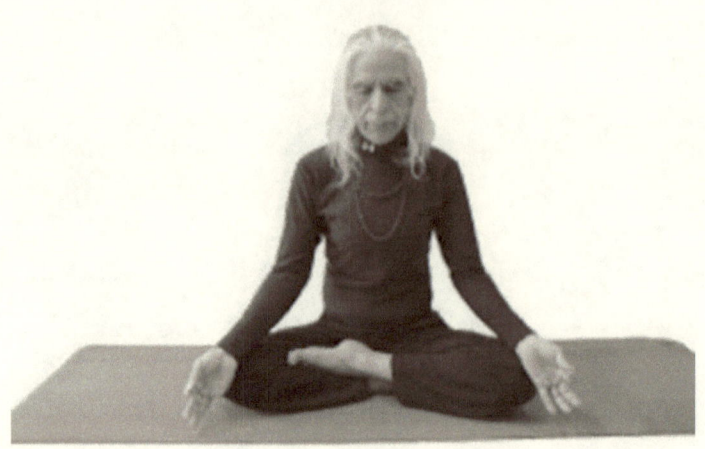

In Sanskrit, 'Siddha' means a spiritually enlightened person. Some praise this posture as even superior to Padmasana for the purpose of Dhyana, or contemplation. It was practiced by many Siddhas, the "perfect yogins" of ancient times; hence the name "Siddhasana'. It brings great purity and holiness.

BENEFITS OF SIDDHASANA

This asana increases digestive fire and gives good appetite, health, and happiness. It removes rheumatism and strengthens the nerves of the legs and thighs. Siddhasana prevents nervous depression from occurring during meditation. It stops the blood pressure from falling too low and also regulates the production of male hormones and helps maintain inner body temperature.

PASCIMOTTANASANA
"Forward bend posture"

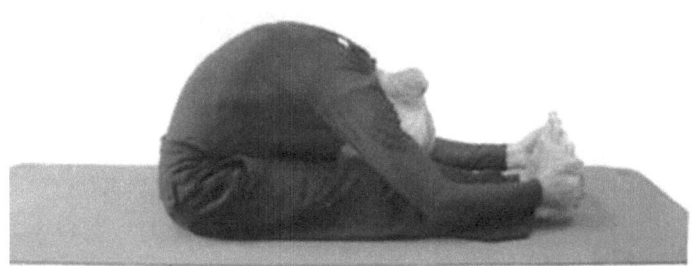

In Sanskrit, *pascima* means west. The back is considered to be the west and the front side to be the east. *Uttana* means stretch out in Sanskrit. *Pascimottanasana* means stretching the back region of the body. With the help of this asana, the dormant forces at the base of spine become active and with regular practice, relaxation deepens.

BENEFITS OF PASCIMOTTASANA

This asana is very useful for dyspepsia, constipation, diabetes, and digestive disorder. It is beneficial for the liver and spleen. It is good for reducing fatty deposits in the abdomen, hips, and thighs. It gives relief in cases of muscular rheumatism of the back. Daily practice of this asana helps to cure impotency and seminal weakness, and increases vitality.

BHUJANGASANA
"Back bend posture"

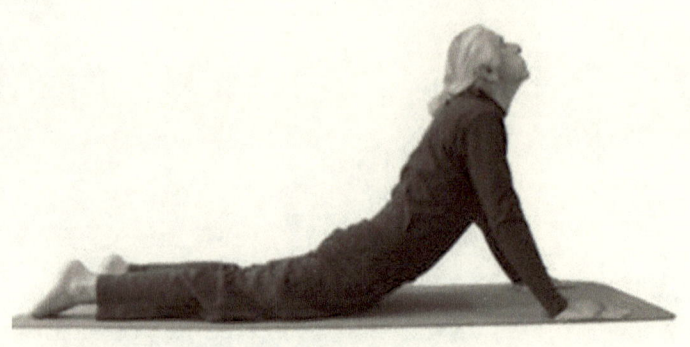

Bhujanga means serpent in Sanskrit. In this posture the body looks like a cobra when it raises its hood. Hence it is called Bhujangasana.

BENEFITS OF BHUJANGASANA

This asana bends the spine backward, which relieves back pain. It increases bodily heat and destroys a host of ailments. Bhujangasana gives a good appetite. Regular practice of this asana relaxes the vertebrae and keeps them in good alignment. This asana strengthens the back, neck, and head. It also expands narrow shoulders and the chest. It gives a gentle massage to the liver, gall bladder, spleen, and pancreas.

SARVANGASANA
"Inverted posture"

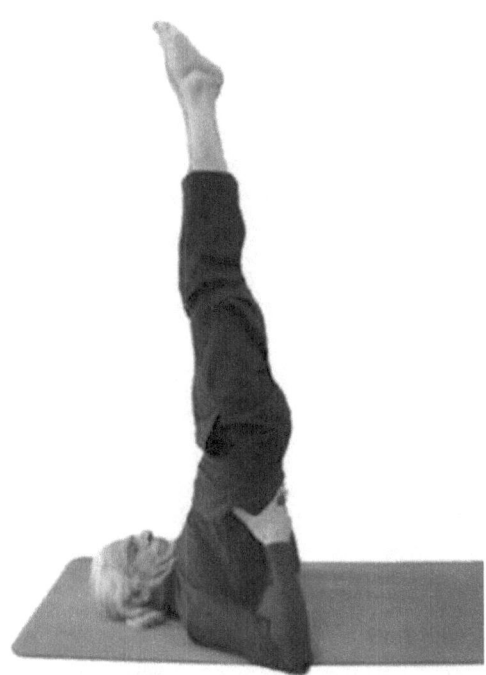

"*Sarva*" means all and *anga* means part in Sanskrit. In this asana, all the parts of the body are engaged. Hence the name Sarvangasana

BENEFITS OF SARVANGASANA

In this asana the thyroid gland is properly nourished. It improves healthy functioning of the circulatory, respiratory, and nervous systems of the body. It supplies a large quantity of blood to the spinal root of nerves. It also keeps the spine quite elastic, which means everlasting youth. It prevents the bones from early hardening and destroys the ravages of old age. Doing this asana regularly strengthens the muscles of the upper arm, shoulders, neck, and thighs.

HALASANA
"Plow Pose"

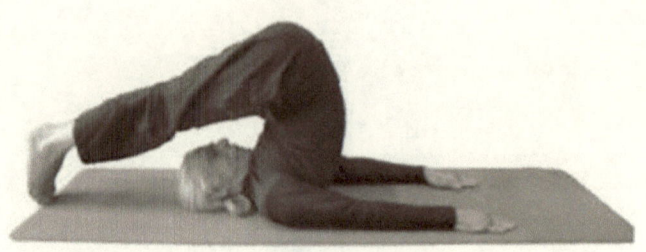

'*Hala*' means plow in Sanskrit. Hence the name Halasana. It replicates the exact appearance of an Indian plow when practiced.

BENEFITS OF HALASANA

This asana helps to maintain abdominal and pelvic organs in their correct positions and strengthens them. It improves digestive power and is conductive to smooth bowel movements. Various sorts of myalgia, sprains, and neuralgias are cured by practicing this asana. This asana also activates, warms up, and lightens the psycho-physiological system.

ARDHA MATSYENDRASANA
"Half twist in a sitting position (1&2)"

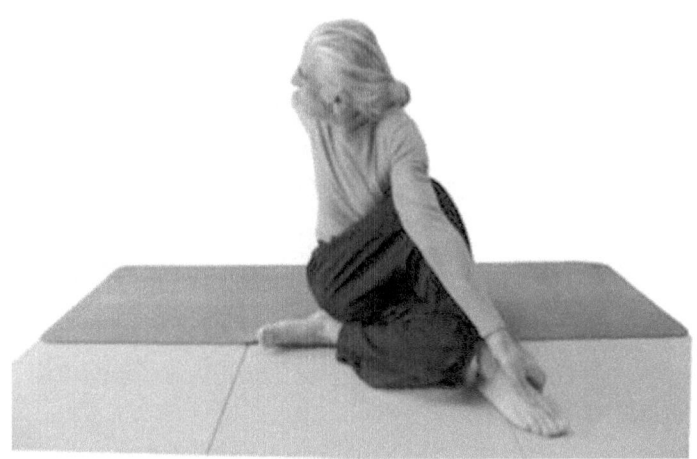

Position 1

Ardha Matsyendrasana is known as the half spinal twist and takes its Sanskrit name from a great yogin named Matsyendra. It translates as the "lord of fish." This asana gives the power that vitalizes and energizes and has the ability to turn on the subtle energies of the body and mind."

ARDHA MATSYENDRASANA
"Half twist in a sitting position"

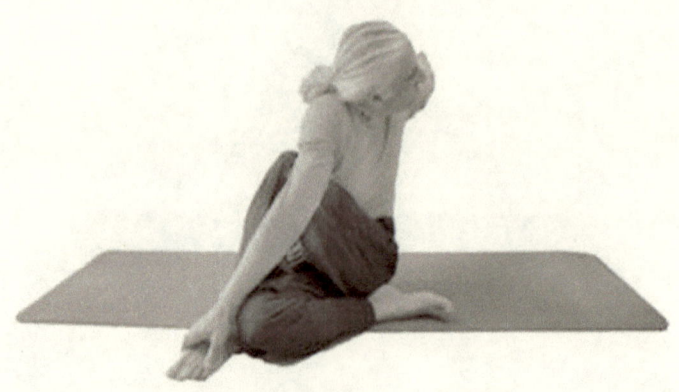

Position 2

BENEFITS OF ARDHA MATSYENDRASANA

This asana is beneficial for diabetes. It increases the capacity of the pancreas and regulates insulin secretion. This asana improves digestion and removes constipation. It is also beneficial for backache. This asana regulates blood circulation around the spine and rotates the spine, making it flexible.

SAVASANA
"The Corpse Pose"

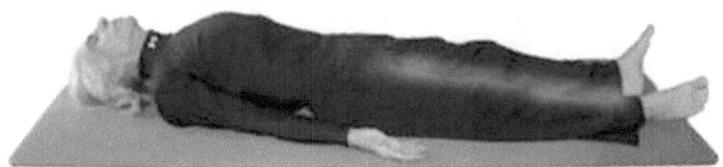

Sava means corpse in Sanskrit. In this asana, the position of the body resembles a corpse. This asana also signifies that one should be dead to external and internal stimulations.

BENEFITS OF SAVASANA

This asana strengthens and tones the entire system. When performing this asana, all the muscles and joints are relaxed. It gives rest not only to the body but also to the mind and soul. Savasana is very useful in managing ailments like hypertension and headaches et cetera. It enhances general well-being. Fits of depression and emotional conflicts are eliminated by the practice of this asana, and inner peace is regained.

PAVAN MUKTASANA
"Leg lock pose"

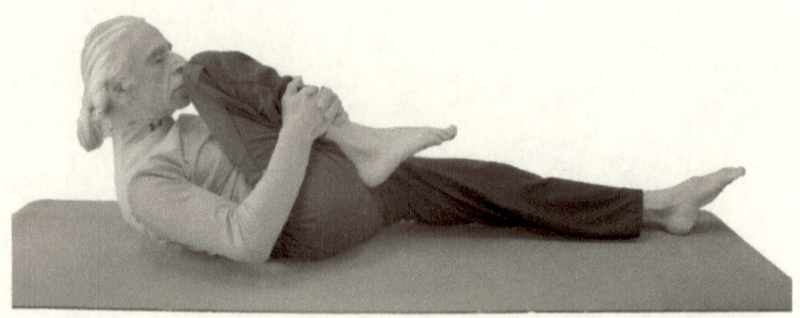

In Sanskrit, *pavana* means wind and *mukta* means release. As the name suggests, this asana massages the digestive organs and gives relief in the stomach and intestines

BENEFITS OF PAVAN MUKTASANA
This asana is beneficial for wind-related stomach problems. It is also beneficial for backache and reduces fat on the stomach.

USTRASANA
"Camel pose"

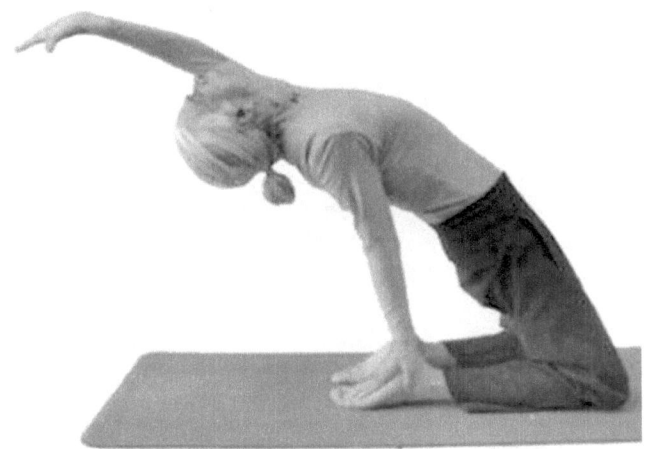

Ustra means camel in Sanskrit. It is also translated as "that which casts light on the mind" and helps release knowledge. The camel revitalizes the mind.

BENEFITS OF USTRASANA

The asana is good for the respiratory system. It is useful for thyroid. This asana cures all the stomach disorders.

UTKATASANA
"Dynamic Energy Pose"

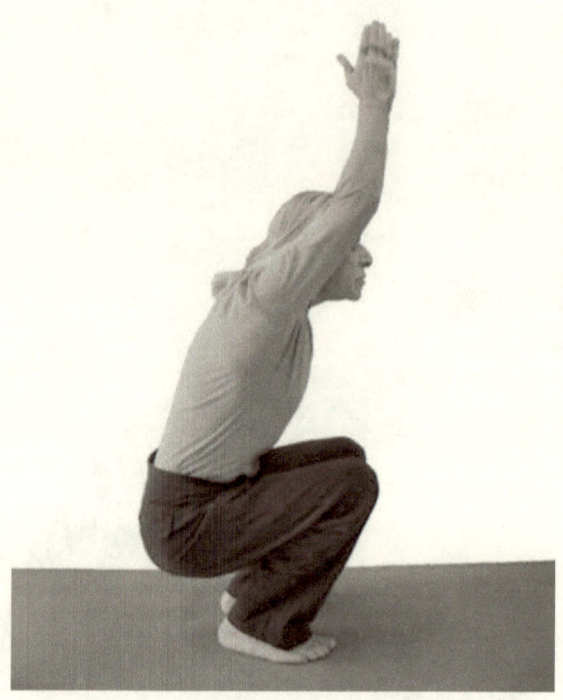

Utkat means powerful, mighty, or uneven. Utkatasana is a posture that forms a zigzag shape with the body, heels, hips, and arms.

BENEFITS OF UTKATASANA

Stretches the Achilles tendon and strengthens the thigh muscles. Strengthens and increases mobility in the ankle, knee, and hip joints.

TRIKONASANA
"Triangle Pose"

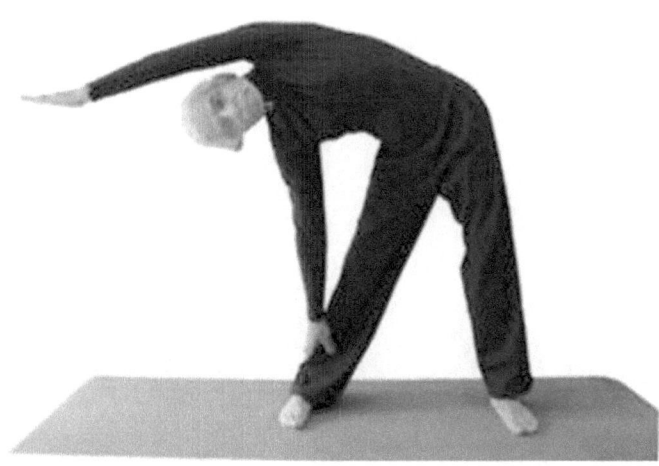

Tri means three, *kona* means angle, and *trikona* means triangle in Sanskrit.

BENEFITS OF TRIKONASANA

Within a few weeks of regular practice of this asana, energy starts flowing to all the muscles of the body. Mentally one feels very energetic. Depression, constipation, and piles are cured.

PADANGUSTHA SPARSASANA
"Single Leg Forward Bend"

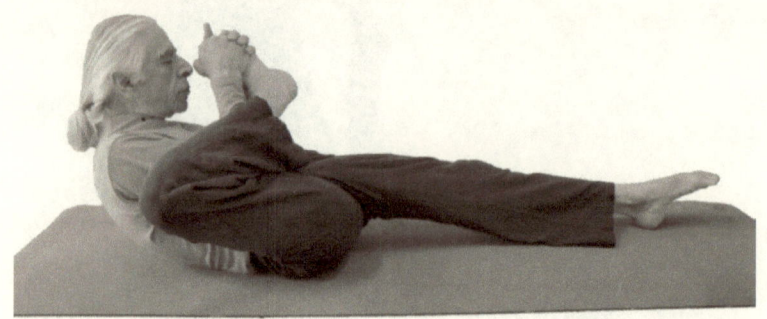

Pada means feet in Sanskrit. In the same way, practice the left leg.

BENEFITS OF PADANGUSTHA SPARSASANA

This asana helps to balance the naval and thus takes care of gas formation, stomach pain, constipation, weakness, and laziness.

SASAKASANA
"The Hare Posture"

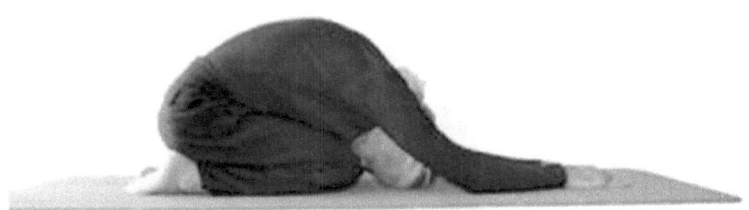

Sasanka means *hare* in Sanskrit. The final position of this asana resembles a hare.

BENEFITS OF SASAKASANA
It massages the heart and is beneficial for heart patients. It gives strength to pancreas, liver, and kidneys.

PARIVRITTA TRIKONASANA
"The Revolving/Reversed Triangle"

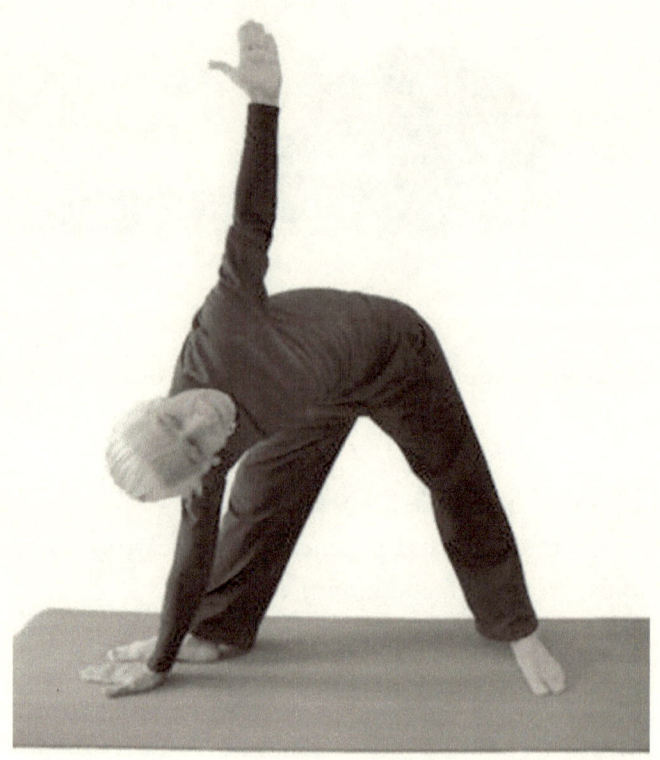

Parivritta means to reserve, and *trikona* means a triangle.

BENEFITS OF PARIVRITTA TRIKONASANA

This asana tones and strengthens the leg muscles. It also increases the blood supply to the back and spinal nerves.

UTTHITA TRIKONASANA
"The Extended Triangle"

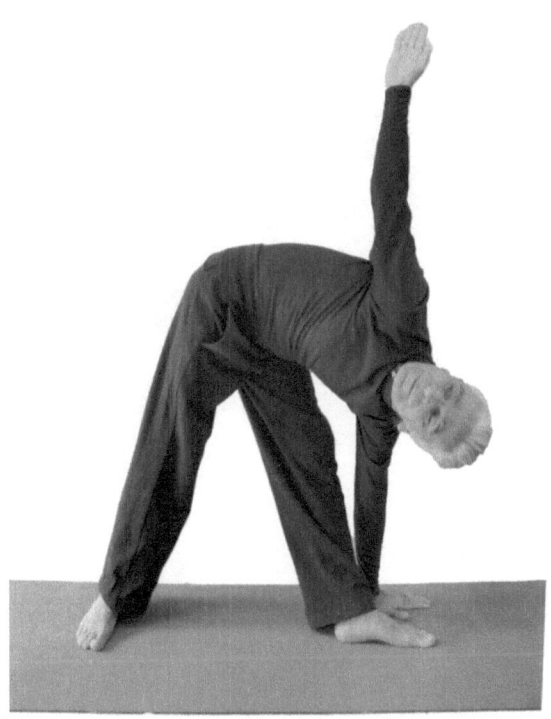

Utthita means extended or stretched, and *trikona* means triangle.

BENEFITS OF UTTHITA TRIKONASANA

This asana helps to remove fat and also tones the leg muscles. It increases hip, shoulder, and leg flexibility.

NAVASANA
"The Boat pose"

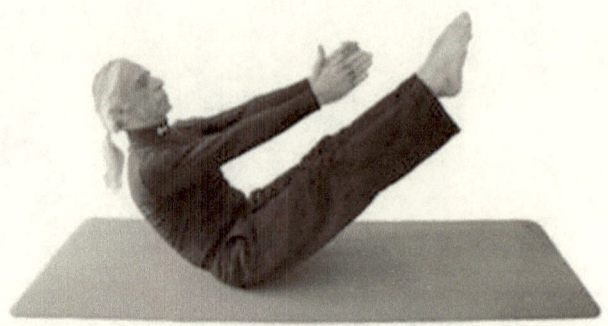

Nava in Sanskrit means a boat. This asana is a balancing pose resembling a boat.

BENEFITS OF NAVASANA
This asana strengthens the muscles of the abdomen, legs, and the back. It also improves balance.

MATSYASANA
"The Fish pose"

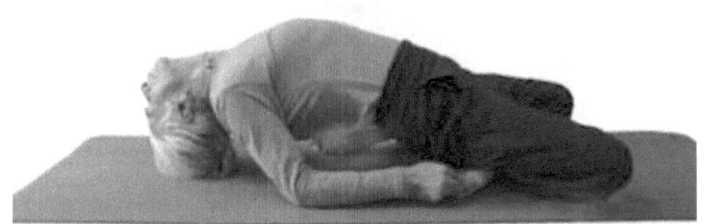

The reason for the name Matsyasana is that, when viewed from above, the body resembles a fish.

BENEFITS OF MATSYASANA

This asana activates the intestines and also makes the thyroid glands healthy.

CHANDRASANA
"The Crescent Moon Pose"

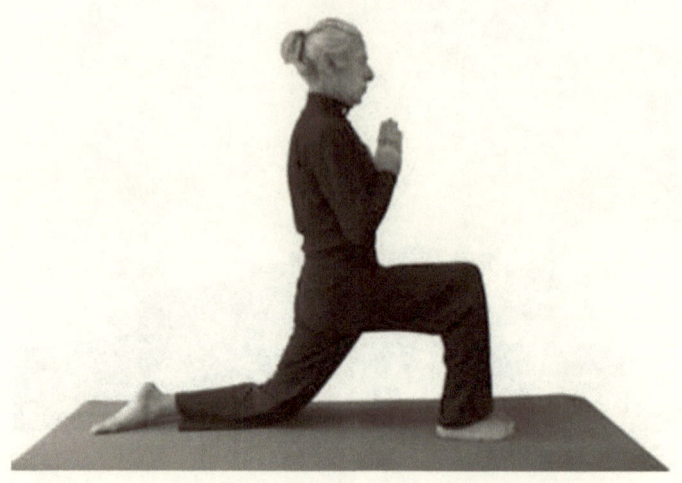

The Crescent Moon and the Pigeon are used as preparatory exercises for hanumanasana (the Splits).

BENEFITS OF CHANDRASANA
This asana increases the blood supply to the pelvic area. It also tones the legs and hips.

PADUNGUSHTASANA
"Celibacy Pose"

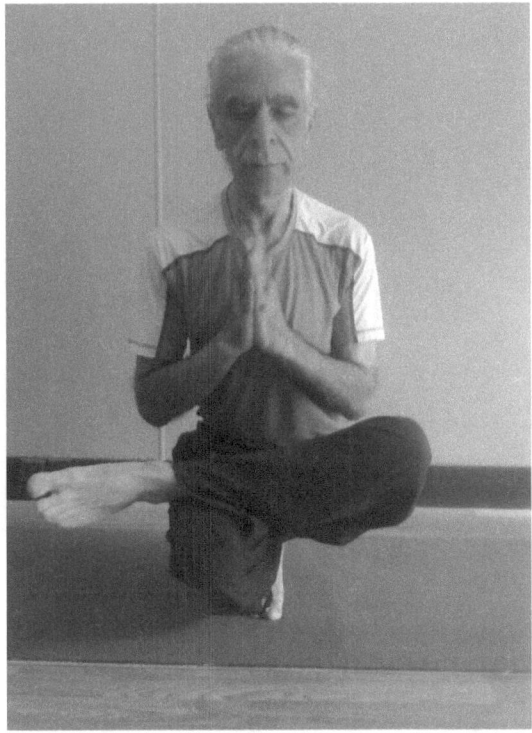

It is useful for celibacy. In Sanskrit *Brahmacharya* is called celibacy.

BENEFITS OF PADUNGUSHTASANA

When practiced for a long time, kundilini awakens and the sperm rises above. It increases strength, intelligence, and vigor.

DHANURASANA
"The Bow pose"

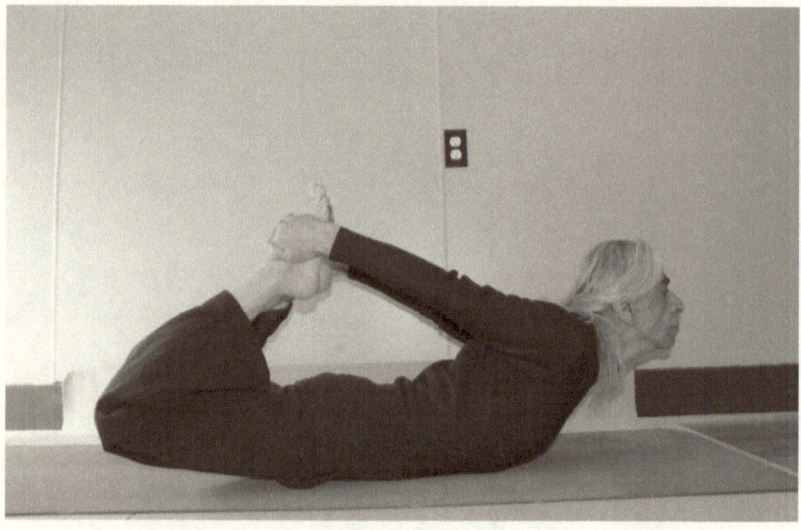

In Sanskrit *Dhanura* means bow.

BENEFITS OF DHANURASANA

It makes the spine strong, healthy, and flexible. It also is beneficial for menstrual-related problems in females. The asana is useful for backaches and stomach pain.

URDHAWATADASANA
"The Mountain pose"

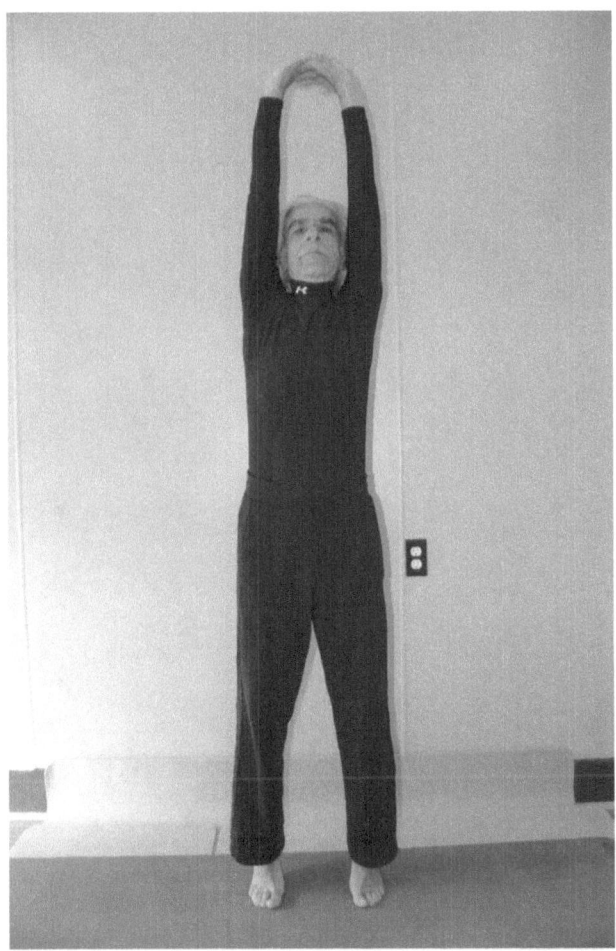

In Sanskrit *Tada* means the pillar.

BENEFITS OF TADASANA.

It cultivates a sense of strength and stability. Tadasana is used as a starting position for almost all the standing postures.

GARUDASANA
"The Eagle pose"

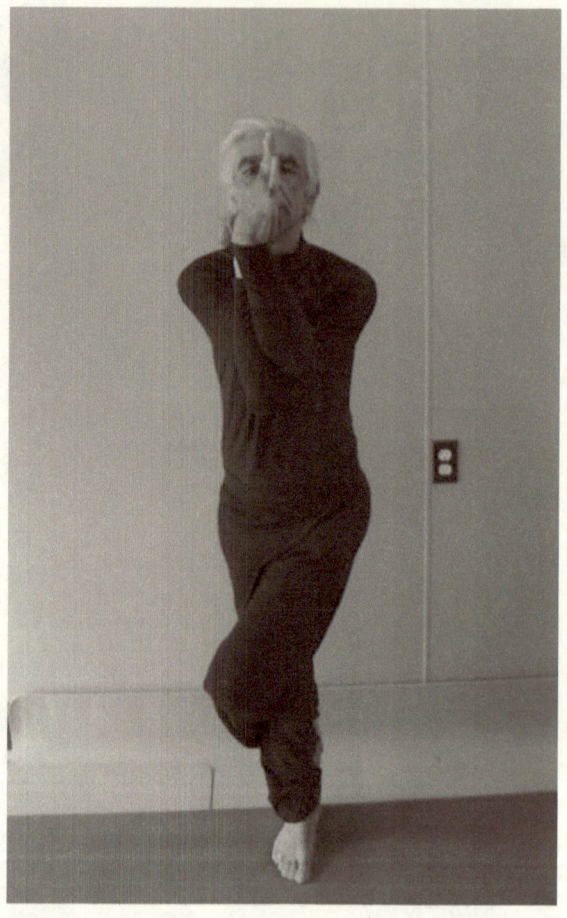

In Sanskrit '*Garuda*' means an eagle. In Indian mythology '*Garuda*' is a deity.

BENEFITS OF GARUDASANA.

This asana is beneficial for hydrosol, male's genital glands, and kidneys. It cures pain in the hands and legs and any other deformity. Also it cures urinary problems.

UTTANASANA
"Standing backward bend"

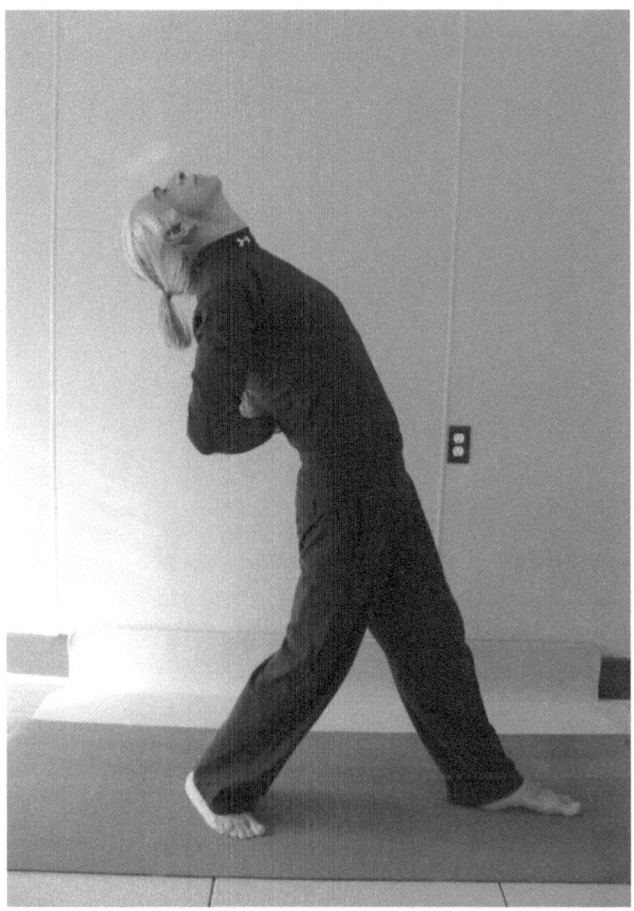

In Sanskrit *Tan* means to stretch or lengthen out and *Ut* refers to an attitude of being deliberate or intense.

BENEFITS OF UTTANASANA.

Gives a gentle massage to the abdominal organs, such as liver and spleen, and also aids digestion.

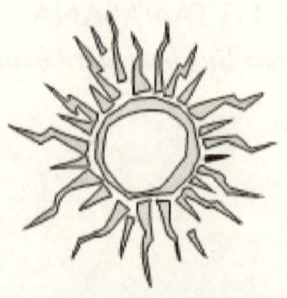

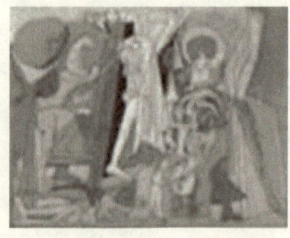

The practice of Asanas is a gateway to the soul. We are able to experience the sense of vitality and joy that yoga practitioners believe is the true nature of the soul.

CHAPTER III

The Sacred Chakras

CHAKRAS

Chakra means wheel in Sanskrit. To heal is to bring the chakras into alignment and balance and awaken them. The chakra as perceived in Indian philosophy does not exist in Western medical science. The framework of chakras is very complex and extensive. It includes the science of the body and knowledge of the nervous system and other energy levels that govern bodily functions.[iv] "Proving" the existence of chakras is similar to "proving" the existence of God.

The earliest known mention of chakras is found in the Upanishads. These Vedic models were adapted into Hinduism and also Tibetan Buddhism as Vajrayana theory, and also the Tantric Shakta theory of chakras. Today, however, there is an increase in awareness and knowledge of chakras in the Western countries, and there is increasing acceptance of the energy centers, at least on some points. There are also models of chakras in other traditions, notably in Chinese and Tibetan Buddhism.

In the spiritual systems of yoga, chakras are thought to be energy nodes within the human body. Manifestation of the cosmic force is expressed through these centers, which energize and govern corresponding regions of the body. The word *chakra* comes from the

Sanskrit and means wheel circle, and sometimes also refers to the wheel of life. In addition to the existing literature in the East on chakras, different Western authors have also tried to describe the chakras, most notably the Theosophists. New Age writers, such as a Danish author and musician Peter Kjaerulff, in his book *The Ring Bearer's Diary* offers insights about the chakras in great detail, including the reasons for their appearance and their functions.

There are also many minor chakras, especially between the major seven chakras. The transpersonal chakra is a chakra that many meditation practitioners say is located above the crown chakra. This chakra is associated with spiritual connection between individuals, as well as connection to the higher consciousness. Parallels have often been drawn by supporters of the existence of chakras between the positions and functions of these chakras and the various organs of the endocrine system.

The seven main chakras are aligned in an ascending column from the base of the spine to the top of the head. Each chakra is associated with a certain color and also associated with multiple specific functions, aspects of consciousness, and other distinguishing characteristics. The seven primary inner chakras from bottom to the top of the humans are as follows:

1. Muladhara Chakra
2. Svadhisthana Chakra
3. Manipura Chakra
4. Anahata Chakra
5. Vishuddha Chakra
6. Ajna or Third Eye Chakra
7. Sahasrara Chakra

These seven chakras are said to reflect how the unified consciousness of a man is divided to manage different aspects of earthly life, namely body instinct, vital energy, deep emotions, communications, and also an overview of life. The chakras are placed at differing levels of spiritual subtlety, with Sahasrara at the top being concerned with pure consciousness and Muladhara at the bottom being concerned with matter.

THE CHAKRAS, THE BODY'S ENERGY CENTERS

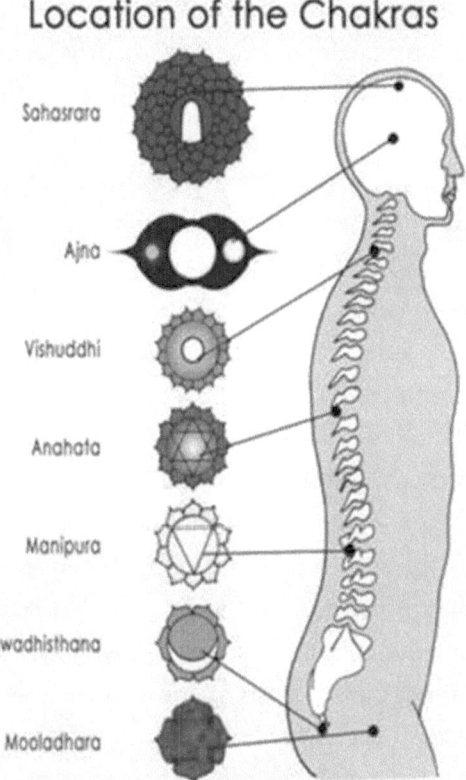

Location of the Chakras

Sahasrara

Ajna

Vishuddhi

Anahata

Manipura

Swadhisthana

Mooladhara

PRANA, OR ENERGY, CENTERS

These chakras are considered sources of life energy, or prana, which is thought to flow among the chakras along pathways called *nadis*. The word *nadi* comes from the Sanskrit root word *nad,* meaning channel, stream, or flow. Prana, or energy, flows and connects the chakras. Nadis are thought to carry a life force energy known as prana in Sanskrit. They are also said to have an extrasensory function, playing a part in empathic and instinctive responses.

The Ida and Pingala nadis are often seen as referring to the two hemispheres of the brain. Pingala is the extroverted solar nadi and corresponds to the left side of the brain. Ida is the introverted lunar nadi and refers to the right side of the brain. The two nadis are stimulated by the practices of pranayama, which involves alternate breathing through left and right nostrils that alternately stimulates the left and right sides of the brain. Sushumna flows inside the central canal of the spinal cord, and Ida and Pingala simultaneously flow on the outer surface of the spinal cord. The chakras are described in the tantric texts as the Sat-Cakra-Nirupana, and also as Padaka-Pancaka, which are described as emanations of consciousness from Brahman, or God.

SAHASRARA CHAKRA

This chakra is positioned above the head or at the top of the head, and it has a thousand petals that are arranged in twenty layers, each of them with fifty petals. This is the abode of Shiva, pure consciousness. Here, the individual consciousness and the cosmic consciousness merge. The Sahasrara, or the crown chakra, is said to be the chakra of consciousness, the master chakra that controls all the others. Its role is very similar to that of the pituitary gland, which secretes hormones to control the rest of the endocrine system. The thalamus is thought to have a key role in the physical basis of consciousness. It is said to be the most subtle chakra in the system, relating to pure consciousness, and it is from this chakra that all the other chakras emanate. When a yogi is able to raise his or her kundalini energy of consciousness up to this point, the state of Samadhi, solace or union with God, is experienced.

Sahasrara Chakra
One thousand petals
Multi-colored lotus'

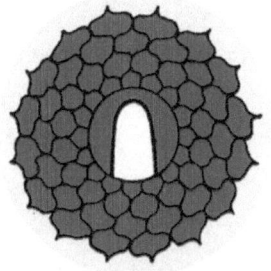

Sahasrara

Sahasrara Chakra

THE AJNA, OR THIRD EYE, CHAKRA

This chakra is the sixth chakra. It is linked to the pineal gland. The point is called Bhrumadhya, where *bhru* means eyebrows and *madhya* means center. It lies between the two eyebrows; this is the place where Indian women put the red dot known as the *tilak*. The eyebrow chakra, namely the Ajna, is the chakra of time and of awareness and light. The pineal gland is light sensitive; it produces the hormone melatonin and regulates going to sleep and awakening. It also produces small amounts of the psychedelic chemical dimethyltryptamine. Awakening this chakra has many physical and mental benefits. It removes mental weakness, increases mental stability, and relaxes the anxious mind. One can also attain inner vision and see all things clearly.

Ajna Chakra
Two petals, silver—gray color lotus

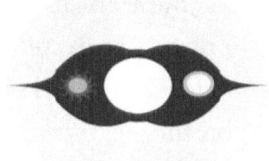

Ajna

Ajna Chakra

VISHUDDHA CHAKRA

This is the throat chakra and is said to be related to communication and growth; it is also the seat of creativity and receptivity. *Vishuddha* means purified. It represents a state of openness in human beings in which life is considered as the provider of experiences and leads to greater understanding. This chakra is parallel to the thyroid gland in the throat and produces thyroid hormone, which is responsible for growth and maturation. Trust, authority, reverence, willingness, and creativity are the qualities related to this chakra. Musicians and artists are said to have their energy concentrated here. This chakra is said to be the legendary fountain of youth.

Visuddha Chakra
'Sixteen petals, violet color lotus

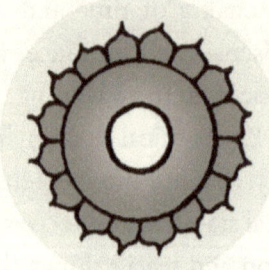

Vishuddhi

Vishuddha Chakra

ANAHATA CHAKRA

This chakra is also known as the heart chakra. It is of great importance and is related to love, equilibrium, possession, power, jealousy, and the well-being of a person. It is related to the thymus located in the chest. The person who meditates on this heart lotus chakra is very wise, and his senses are completely under control. This chakra, if awakened, can fulfill wishes; it has the power to allow a person to preordain his fate, allowing the person to create his or her own destiny. This chakra is also a part of the immune system, as well being part of the endocrine system. It produces T cells responsible for fighting off disease and is adversely affected by stress.

Anahata Chakra
Twelve petals, blue color lotus

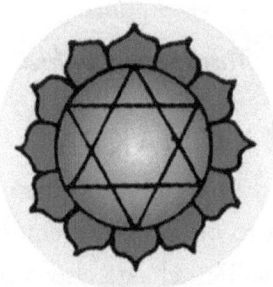

Anahata

Anahata Chakra

MANIPURA CHAKRA

The solar plexus Manipura chakra is derived from two Sanskrit words: *mani*, meaning jewel, and *pura*, meaning city. Therefore, the chakra means the city of jewel. When this chakra is awakened, it is responsible for the strong willpower in a human being and a desire for high achievement in the life span of a person. It is located directly behind the navel on the inner wall of the spinal column. It is related to energy, assimilation, and digestion and is said to correspond to the roles played by the pancreas and the outer adrenal glands, the adrenal cortex. These play a valuable role in digestion, the conversion of food matter into energy for the body. It is said that meditation on this chakra leads to the knowledge of the entire physical system. and the body becomes disease free.

Manipura Chakra
Ten petals, bright yellow color lotus

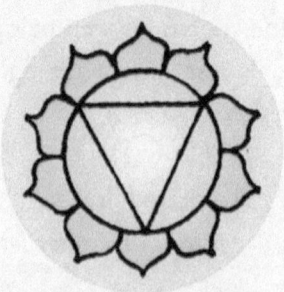

Manipura

Manipura Chakra

SVADHISTHANA CHAKRA

This chakra is located in the groin at the termination of the spinal cord. This chakra is said to be related to emotion, sexuality, creativity, social, ambition, et cetera. This chakra also corresponds to the testes or the ovaries, which produce the various sex hormones involved in the reproductive cycle and which can cause dramatic mood swings. It is said that all the experiences and karmas of the past lives of which a person is mostly unconscious in the present life are symbolized in the Svadhisthana chakra. Many instinctive drives that we now and then experience simmer up from this chakra, of which most of us are usually unaware.

Svadhisthana Chakra
Six petal, vermilion color lotus

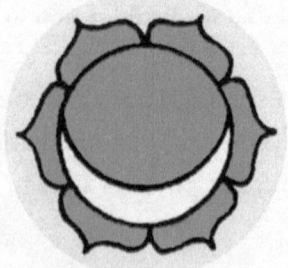

Swadhisthana

Swadhisthana Chakra

MULADHARA CHAKRA

This chakra is positioned close to the anus, at the perineum; it has four petals that match the *vritti* of the greatest joy, natural pleasure, delight in controlling passion, and blissfulness in concentration. According to the Sankhya philosophy, the concept of Muladhara is that of *moola prakriti*, a metaphysical basis of the material existence. Muladhara is the chakra that draws down spiritual energy and causes it to assume a physical existence. Within this chakra resides or sleeps the kundalini Shakti, the great spiritual potential waiting to be aroused and brought back up to the source from which it originated: the Brahman, or absolute. Muladhara is the base from which the three main psychic nadis emerge, namely Ida, Pingala, and Sushumna. This chakra is also related to the physical processes of reproduction and excretion and to the various fear and guilt complexes associated with them. All of the human Samskaras (potential karmas) are expressed here in a physical form.

This chakra is associated with the Vedic deities, like Indra and Brahma. Its element is Earth, and the color is red. The energy called the Kundalini that was unleashed in creation lies coiled and sleeping, and it is the purpose of a tantric yogi to arouse this energy and cause it to rise up through the increasingly subtler chakras until union with God is achieved in the Sahasrara chakra at the crown of the head. This union is the highest, according to the Tantric literature. When a yogi is able to achieve this union, he becomes fully aware and achieves enlightenment.

Mooladhara Chakra
Four petals, deep red color lotus

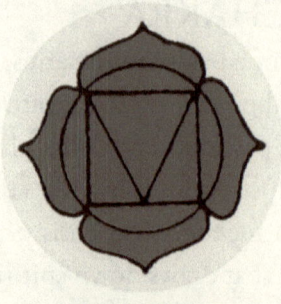

Mooladhara

Mooladhara Chakra

CHAKROLOGY

There are many different chakrologies, most of them based on the Vedic esoteric interpretations of the Tantric Shakti; the ancient Greeks and some Europeans also contributed to it. A Croatian esoteric philosopher and physicist Arvan Harvat noticed that it would be very difficult to develop a unified coherent chakra science that would integrate all the elements of the various present chakrologies.

Although there is no evidence that Indian mystics made this association themselves, it is noted by many that there is a marked similarity between the positions and roles described for chakras and the positions and roles of the glands in the endocrine system and also by the positions of the nerve ganglia, also known as plexuses, along the spinal column, opening the possibility that two vastly different systems of conceptualization have been brought to bear to systemize insights about the same phenomenon. Chakras are thought of as having their physical manifestation in the body as these glands and their subjective manifestation as the associated psychological and spiritual experiences.

SEVEN MAJOR SACRED CHAKRAS

Names of the chakras	Position of chakras	Type Personality	Number of petals of chakras	Element of chakras
Sahasrara	Top of the head	Primordial Imagination Understanding Cosmic Consciousness	One thousand petals (infinite) Multicolor or red lotus	
Ajna	Middle of forehead	Intuitive Visionary type	Two petals Silver-Gray lotus	
Vishuddha	Throat	Communication Creativity Contemplative	Sixteen petals Violet color lotus	Earth
Anahata	Center of chest	Self-centered Love, Hope Compassion	Twelve petals Blue color lotus	Air
Manipura	Solar Plexus	Intellectual Energy, Vitality Desire & Power	Ten petals Bright yellow lotus	Fire

Svadhisthanna	Splenic Plexus	Social-gregarious Ambition, Intimacy	Six petals Vermilion color lotus	Water
Muladhara	Base of Spine	Physical-Sensation Survival	Four petals Deep red.	Earth

CHAPTER IV

Pranayama: The Art of Yoga Breathing

PRANAYAMA

Pranayama is a method of controlling prana, or the life force, through the regulation of breathing. Sage Patanjali says that retention of breath after expiration removes the obstacles to yoga. According to Hatha Yoga Pradipika, only when the body is flexible from performing various asanas and when you have control of the body through a balanced diet, only then should pranayama be practiced.

The breath is divided into three phases:

1. **Puraka** (inhalation)
2. **Rechaka** (exhalation)
3. **Kumbhaka** (retention of the breath)[2]

Prana and mind are intricately linked; fluctuation of one leads to the fluctuation of the other. When either the mind or the prana is balanced, it leads to the balance of the other. The practice of Hatha Yoga controls the prana and the mind automatically, whereas Raja Yoga

---

[2]   These are discussed in more detail later in this chapter.

controls the mind; thereby the prana becomes controlled. These are two paths leading to the art of yoga breathing.

In pranayma, it is the duration of the breath retention that is increased. When retention is held for a prolonged period, mental agitation is calmed. As long as the vayu, or air, or prana remains in the body, that is called life. Therefore it is necessary to retain vayu. During breath retention, the two poles of energy come closer together. It is necessary to try to lead a peaceful life; thereby the mind remains controlled.

To breathe is to live, and without breath there is no life. All forms of animals, higher or lower in form, breathe to live. In a normal state there is no need for instructions in breathing. However, the percentage of humans who breathe correctly is very small.

For success in the practices of pranayama, it is necessary to free the mind from untruthfulness, ignorance, and all other painful and unpleasant experiences of the body and mind; the mind thus becomes clean, and it becomes easy for the student to concentrate on the desired object. It becomes possible for him to progress further in the direction of Dhyana Yoga and Samadhi.

Physically, pranayama appears to be a systematic exercise of respiration, which makes the lungs stronger, improves blood circulation, makes the person healthier, and bestows upon him or her the boon of a long life. Physiology teaches us that the air, or prana, we breathe in fills our lungs and spreads throughout the entire body, providing it with essentials, taking them to the heart and then to the lungs, which then expels useless material like carbon dioxide out of the body through the act of exhalation. If respiratory exercise is done regularly and efficiently, lungs become stronger, and the blood becomes pure and clean.

The ultimate purpose of life is attained, according to Bhagavad Gita and Upanishads, by taking a path toward God. The ancient yogis who lived in the forests discovered that the life span of every living creature was determined according to their respiration. Tortoises and elephants take approximately four breaths per minute and live about three hundred years. The yogis realized that the same principle could be applied to human beings. Man breathes fifteen to eighteen times per minute, or 21,600 times in a twenty-four hour period; humans live, on average, seventy-five to a hundred years. By slowing down the breath and taking long and deep respirations, according to the ancient yogis we can increase the span of our lives. In times of stress, anger, and mental anxiety, the rate of breathing generally increases; thereby the longevity of our life decreases. We are usually unaware of this connection between respiration and mind. If our mind is unstable, we are subject to sickness, and we are able to hold our breath only for a short while. Under normal conditions, nature dictates that cells in the body must gradually decay and die, but the yogis who do a lot of pranayama recharge and magnetize their cells.

A long breath increases the ability to concentrate, while simultaneously increasing the life span. The yogis realized the importance of an adequate oxygen supply thousands of years ago; that is why they developed and perfected various breathing techniques that helped them to revitalize their minds and their bodies and increased the length of their life span.

One of the five principles of yoga is pranayama, or breathing exercise. From the yogic point of view, proper breathing brings more oxygen to the blood and to the brain. Pranayama also goes hand in hand with the yoga asanas. The union of these two yogic practices is considered the highest form of purification and self-discipline, covering both mind and body. These techniques have also proved to increase prevention of major diseases and to cure some illnesses.

BREATHING IS IMPORTANT FOR TWO REASONS

- It is the only means of supplying our bodies and its various organs with oxygen, which is vital for our life.
- It is one of the ways to get rid of waste products and toxins from our body.

THE FIVE PRANAS

According to the philosophy of yoga, our physical body has two types of energies. One is known as vital or dynamic energy, and the other is known as manas or chitt-shakti, or mental, energy. Through the nadis, or channels, there is the flow of consciousness. These two systems are interconnected within the body; thereby every organ is supplied with mental and pranic energy. It is estimated that there are about 72,000 nadis, which cover the whole body and through which prana and consciousness are distributed through the body. Out of these nadis, three are the most important. These are Ida, Pingala, and Sushumna. Ida nadi is the channel for mental energy; it is also known as the moon. Pingala nadi is the channel for vital energy, also known as the sun. Sushumna nadi is the channel for awakening of spiritual consciousness. These three nadis are known as pranic force, mental force, and the spiritual force. They originate at the Muladhara Chakra, which is situated in the perineum.

According to yoga, the pranic body which comprise of the individual prana and a network of nadis which carry the prana, is divided into five forms, collectively they are known as the Pancha pranas; these pranic clouds are free to expand or contract with or without the influence of any external factor.

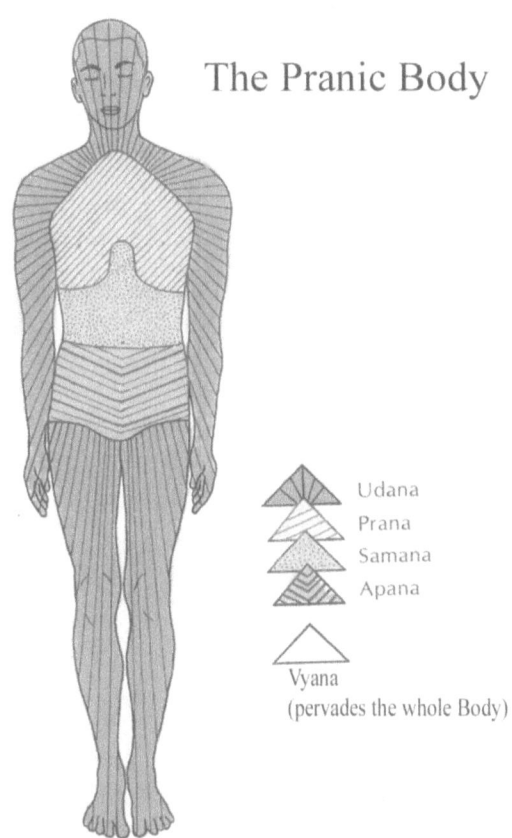

Structure of the five Pranas in the Body

THE FIVE FORMS OF PRANA

1. UDANA-VAYU

Corresponds to the throat region and is the function of speech. Udana regulates the processes of acceptance and absorption of desired elements in the body. It is the source of activation of the Vishuddhi Chakra.

2. PRANA-VAYU

Corresponds to the chest region. This sub-prana is not the overall prana here but belongs to a specific part of the body between the larynx and the

103

top of the diaphragm. It controls the functioning of the heart and lungs and is the source of respiration. It is associated with the Anahata Chakra.

3. SAMANA-VAYU

Corresponds to the central region of the body and is located between the navel and the ribcage. Between the two opposite forces of prana and apana, it acts as an equalizer for these forces. It is responsible for the digestion and assimilation of nutrients. Samana activates the metabolic process and is regarded as the source of power in the Manipura Chakra.

4. APANA-VAYU

Corresponds to the region of the lower abdomen that is located in the pelvic region, between the navel and the perineum. It controls the function of the kidneys, bladder, bowels, and the excretory and reproductive organs.

5. VYANA-VAYU

Corresponds to distribution of energy to all the areas of the body. Vyana regulates blood circulation and is described as the source of power for the Svadhishthana Chakra.

In addition to the five major pranas, there are five other small pranas, such as naga, which is responsible for belching and hiccupping. Korma opens the eyes, krkara induces hunger and thirst in living beings; devadatta is responsible for yawning, and dhananjaya is responsible for decomposition of the body after death.

OXYGEN IS VITAL FOR OUR BODIES

OXYGEN IS THE MOST VITAL NUTRIENT IN OUR BODIES.

- It is essential for the proper and efficient functioning of the brain, nerves, glands, and other internal organs.

- We can survive without food for weeks and without water for days, but without oxygen we will die within a few minutes.
- If the brain does not get a proper supply of this essential nutrient, it will cause degradation of all the vital organs of the body.
- The brain requires more oxygen than any other organ. If it doesn't get enough, the result is mental sluggishness, negative thoughts, depression, and, eventually, declines in vision and hearing.

OXYGEN PURIFIES THE BLOODSTREAM

One of the major secrets of energy and rejuvenation is a purified blood stream. The quickest and most effective way to purify the blood stream is by taking in extra supplies of oxygen from the air we breathe. The breathing exercises described below are the most effective methods ever devised for saturating the blood with extra oxygen.

Breathing, which is usually thought of as merely a single inhalation followed by a single exhalation, can be analyzed into four phases or stages, each with its distinct nature and traditional Sanskrit name. The transitions from inhaling to exhaling and from exhaling to inhaling involve reversals in the direction of the movements of muscles and of expansive or contractive movements of lungs, thorax, and abdomen. The time necessary for such reversals can be very short, as may be observed if one deliberately pants as shortly and rapidly as he can. Yet they can be long, as one may notice if he intentionally stops breathing when he has finished in-breathing or out-breathing. The effects of these pauses, especially when they are lengthened, may be deliberate at first and then seem remarkably spontaneous.

FOUR STAGES OF BREATHING

1. PURAKA (INHALATION)

A single inhalation is termed puraka. Inhalation is the active process of drawing in air and requires muscular effort to draw air into the lungs. The inhalation is expected to be smooth and continuous. If a person should pause one or more times during the process of a single inhaling, the process might be spoken of as a broken puraka.

2. ABHYANTARA KUMBHAKA

Kumbhaka means breath retention. There are two types: *sahita kumbhaka*, which is deliberately holding the breath, or *kevala kumbhaka*, where the breath becomes suspended automatically. Kumbhaka also refers to the suspension of the breath as a part of pranayama practices. The main effect of kumbhaka is to train the nervous system to tolerate higher levels of carbon dioxide in the body. The aim of all pranayama practices is to achieve kevala kumbhaka, which is the stage of samadhi. Deprived of oxygen, the human organs and cells cease to function while remaining preserved until the yogi chooses to reactivate himself. This practice of kumbhak must be undertaken only under the guidance of a very experienced teacher.

3. RECHAKA (EXHALATION)

The third stage exhalation is called recaka. Like inhalation, it too should be smooth and continuous, though often the speed of exhaling is different from that of inhaling. Normally, muscular energy is used for inhaling, whereas exhaling consists merely of relaxing the tensed muscles. Such relaxing forces air from the lungs as they return to a relaxed condition. Muscular effort may also be used for both inhalation and exhalation. You can force air out with muscular effort, like when you sit or stand erect with your abdominal muscles under constant control. When you deliberately smooth the course of breathing and hold the cycle in regular or irregular patterns, you are also likely to use muscular energy at each stage, including the pauses. However, in a condition of complete relaxation, you should expect to exert some effort for inhalation.

4. BAHYA KUMBHAKA (PAUSE AFTER EXHALING)

The fourth stage of breathing, the pause after exhaling, is also called kumbhaka, especially when the stoppage is deliberate or automatically prolonged. This empty pause completes the cycle, which terminates as the pause ends and a new inhalation begins.

Good health, efficient respiratory function, and increased vitality are only the foundations for the more advanced practices that involve kumbhaka.

Prana vidya can be used to consciously manipulate and improve personal health. In prana vidya, the knowledge of prana and the ability, through this knowledge, to manipulate it, the practitioner extracts the life force, or essence, and sends it to the various parts of the body. Benefits of prana vidya are felt at three levels: physical, psychological, and spiritual. First, however, the mastery of prana techniques is required before the benefits can be derived. Physical benefits are better functioning of all the inner organs, including circulation. The psychological benefit is complete rejuvenation of the body. Because of the practice of prana vidya, our state of mind attains a higher state of consciousness. The dormant centers of the personality respond to the will, and you learn how to use the subconscious and unconscious minds. Therefore, prana vidya involves the awakening of the total personality and leads to emancipation.

Prana vidya is a very powerful technique, and therefore it is recommended that a beginner prepare adequately. If possible, training should be taken under an expert guidance.

THE TECHNIQUES OF PRANAYAMA

As this is not a book on pranayama, only the most basic and helpful pranayama techniques are provided. For beginners, it's a good place to start with these techniques.

KAPALBHATI (THE CLEANSING BREATH)

This breathing technique is used specifically for cleansing. The practice cleanses the nasal passages in the skull and other passages of the respiratory system. If you have a lot of mucus in the air passages or feel tension and blockages in the chest, it is often helpful to breathe quickly. This section we will introduce you to this breathing technique and point out its benefits.

In Kapalabhati, the breath is short, rapid, and strong. We use the lungs as a pump, creating so much pressure as they expel the air that all the waste is removed from the air passages and from the lungs up through the nostrils. *Kapala* means forehead, and *bhati* means that which brings lightness. Kapalabhati is a good to practice when we feel heavy or foggy in the head. If we have problems with the sinuses or feel numb around the eyes, Kapalabhati invigorates the entire brain. Here, only Vatakrama Kapalbhati is explained. In Kapalbhati, greater numbers of respirations can be taken than in bhastrika pranayama, which is covered in depth later in this section, because hyperventilation does not occur.

KAPALBHATI TECHNIQUE 1

1. Sit in a comfortable meditative pose: Padmasana or Siddhasana.
2. Place your hands on the knees.
3. Close your eyes, keeping the spine erect.
4. Inhale deeply and perform 20 to 30 fast respirations through both nostrils, placing more emphasis on exhalation. Inhalation is to be short.
5. After the last exhalation, inhale deeply through the nose and exhale quickly through the mouth.
6. On completion, sit quietly for a minute or two.

ANTAR KUMBHAKA TECHNIQUE 2

1. Practice 30 to 40 Kapalbhati breaths as per the above method.
2. Upon completion of the last exhalation, breathe in fully, hold your breath as long as comfortably possible.
3. Then exhale completely from your nostrils.
4. After few normal breaths, begin the next round.

BENEFITS

Kapalabhati flushes out stale residual air in the lungs and helps a fresh supply of air to reach the lungs. It lends elasticity to the diaphragm and increases the capacity of the lungs. This practice is very helpful for those who suffer from asthma, emphysema, and bronchitis

We must be very careful with these techniques because there is a danger of creating tension in the breath. We may also become dizzy when we breathe rapidly; for this reason we always conclude the practice of Kapalabhati with some slow breaths. It is important not to breathe rapidly too many times. After a few rapid breaths, take several slow ones and emphasize the long exhalation.

BHASTRIKA PRANAYAMA

Bhastrika means bellows in Sanskrit. Just as a blacksmith works his bellows, in the same way the abdominal muscles are exercised during the practice of Bhastrika, in which air is forcefully drawn in and pushed out. Bhastrika Pranayama is a combination of Kapalabhati and Ujjayi Pranayama.

PRELIMINARY METHOD TECHNIQUE 1

1. Sit in Padamasana position or any meditative pose, erect and comfortable.
2. Keep neck and abdomen in alignment.
3. Practice Kapal Bhati vigorously 20 to 30 times, as suits your lung capacity.
4. After the last exhalation of breath, empty the lungs completely and inhale as slowly and deeply as possible through both nostrils to the full capacity of the lungs, while expanding the lungs slowly and naturally and keeping the abdominal muscles controlled. Breathe out forcefully, without strain, through the nose.
5. One breath in and one breath out taken together, completes one circuit of bastrika. Complete 5 to 7 of these circuits at a stretch to complete one cycle.

6. End the process with usual breathing. End the process and come to the state as of usually breathing

Bhastrika primarily consists of forced, rapid, deep breathing; it serves as a basis for many varieties of exercises, all of which may be described by the same name. Although air is forced both in and out, the emphasis is placed upon the expulsion of the air. A series of such expulsions, each following the other in quick succession without either full or empty pause, is called *a round*. Beginners should limit a round to about ten exhalations, though the number may be slowly increased if desired.

BASIC METHOD TECHNIQUE 2

1. Sit comfortably in a meditative asana.
2. Close the right nostril with the right thumb.
3. Breathe in and out forcefully through the left nostril about 10 to 15 times; do not strain. After completion take a deep breath in and out of the left nostril.
4. Close the left nostril and breathe in and out forcefully 10 to 15 times through the right nostril.
5. After completion, take a deep breath in and out through the right nostril.
6. Release the nasikagra mudra and place the hands on the knees. Perform rapid inhalation and exhalation through both the nostrils together.
7. This is one round, consisting of using the left and right and both nostrils together.

ANTARA KUMBHAKA TECHNIQUE 3

1. Start bhastrika in the left nostril and complete 15 rounds.
2. Inhale deeply through the left nostril, close both nostrils, and hold the breath inside for a few seconds or as long as you can

comfortably retain your breath. Then exhale through your left nostril.

3. Close the left nostril with your thumb, keeping the right nostril open.
4. Take 15 rapid breaths through the right nostril.
5. Then inhale fully through the right nostril, and hold the breath for few seconds.
6. Exhale through the right nostril; release nasikagra mudra
7. Practice 15 times through both nostrils.
8. After the last exhalation, inhale fully through both nostrils and then hold the breath in kumbhaka until uncomfortable; then exhale through both nostrils.
9. Allow the breath to return to normal before continuing.
10. Start with three rounds and slowly increase; do not strain.

ANULOMA VILOMA

This technique is also called Alternate Nostril Breathing. *Anuloma* means toward, and *viloma* means reverse in Sanskrit. In this breathing technique, you inhale through one nostril, retain the breath, and exhale through the other nostril in a ratio of 2:8:4. The left nostril is the path of the nadi called Ida, and the right nostril is the path of the nadi called Pingala. If you are really healthy, you will breathe predominantly through the Ida nostril about one hour and fifty minutes, then through the Pingala nostril. But in many people, this natural rhythm is disturbed. Anuloma Viloma restores, equalizes, and balances the flow of prana in the body. One round of Anuloma Viloma is made up of six steps, as shown below. Start by practicing three rounds and build up slowly to twenty rounds, extending the count within the given ratio.

ANULOMA VILOMA (ALTERNATE NOSTRIL BREATHING)

1. Inhale through the left nostril, closing the right with the thumb, to the count of four.
2. Hold the breath, closing both nostrils, to the count of sixteen.
3. Exhale through the right nostril, closing the left with the ring and little fingers, to the count of eight.
4. Inhale through the right nostril, keeping the left nostril closed with the ring and little fingers, to the count of four.
5. Hold the breath, closing both nostrils, to the count of sixteen
6. Exhale through the left nostril, keeping the right closed with the thumb, to the count of eight.
7. Take a normal respiration between each round
8. Practice 10 rounds

BENEFITS OF ANULOMA VILOMA

The exercise of the Anuloma Viloma produces optimum function to both sides of the brain: that is, optimum creativity and optimum logical and verbal activity. This will make both sides of the brain—the left side, which is responsible for logical thinking, and the right side, which is responsible for creative thinking—to function properly. This will lead to a balance between a person's creative and logical thinking. The yogis consider this to be the best technique to calm the mind.

Doing pranayama does not simply mean taking air into the body and throwing it out; along with oxygen we also take in vital energy. Pranayama is also a path to build a link with the Supreme power.

RULES FOR PRANAYAMA

- Select a peaceful and a clean place for pranayma in a well-ventilated place, or outdoors.
- Breathe only through the nose, as the air is then filtered.

- Practice pranayma on an empty stomach in the morning or three to four hours after eating.
- Keep the mind calm and composed while performing pranayma
- Practice of pranayma should be performed slowly; the timeframe for pranayma should be gradually increased
- Most important in pranayma is the daily routine and a disciplined lifestyle.

CHAPTER V

Yoga and Ayurveda

AYURVEDA

The word *Ayurveda* is made up of two words: *Ayu*, meaning life, and *Veda*, meaning knowledge, wisdom, or essential truth. Ayurveda means knowledge of life. It is this principle of life that is applied to holistic health, harmony, and happiness; though a system of medicine, it aims at knowing one's essential nature. Ayurveda is a system of diet, healing, and health maintenance and is the oldest science of life, just like the science of yoga. Ayurveda combines yoga, meditation, food, cleansing, and regenerative treatments. The science of Ayurveda divides the human body into three basic components: Dosha, Dhatu, and Mala.

These are also said to be composed of the five elements and are linked to each other and are influenced by the external environment. The main pillar of the human organism is the troika (i.e., Dosha, Dhatu and Mala) along with Agni, the fire of life. The fourth component is the mind; it is a most important component, according to Ayurveda. The spirit is also considered an important component of the body.

The troika should be in harmony, with all the components properly balanced. The overall effect is physical strength, better health, inner peace, and calmness. According to Ayurveda, life is a combination of senses, mind, body, and soul. It teaches us to understand our body and our particular nature at a deep physical, mental, and emotional level. With that knowledge we are able to identify activities, conditions, and foods to keep us healthy and in balance. Ayurvedic principles are utilized not only to treat persons who are ill but also to prepare a balanced meal and a constant harmonious environment.

BASIC PRINCIPLES OF AYURVEDA

I.   The five universal elements, or *Pancha mahabhutas*, form the physiology of Ayurveda.

II. Body constitution in Ayurveda

III. Seven steps of physiology: Sapta Dhatus

IV. Treatment of disease: Samprapti

The functioning of our body and its tendencies are directly related to five elements, which act as the basic energies in everybody and everything. Sattva is the power of harmony and balance. Rajas is the power of energy, action, and movement. Tamas is the power of darkness, the physical matter.

FIVE UNIVERSAL ELEMENTS: PANCHA MAHABHUTAS

According to Ayurveda, we should think about which of the five elements—space, air, fire, water and earth—seem to be strongest in our personalities. According to the science of Ayurveda, there are different combinations of the great elements of which we are constituted. Space and air constitute Vata. Fire and water constitute Pitta. Water and earth constitute Kapha. These three doshas, or humors, govern the biological and psychological processes in our body, mind, and consciousness.

These elements get combined in varieties such that each form of matter is distinctly unique. They constantly change and interact with each other, which keeps the world going. All this happens under the influence of the modes, or the gunas.

In the case of a human being, for instance, space corresponds to the spaces within the body (mouth, nostrils, et cetera); air denotes the movement (muscular or nervous system also); fire controls the functioning of enzymes (intelligence and digestive system); water is in all body fluids (saliva and digestive juices); earth manifests in the solid structures of the body (bones, teeth, flesh, and hair). Following is the relationship of the five elements with the sense organs:

Space—> Sound
Air—> Touch
Fire—> Sight
Water—> Taste
Earth—> Smell

The Human Constitution: space, air, fire, water, and earth are the five basic elements that constitute a human body. The physical body is formed by the transaction of five basic elements into doshas.

DOSHAS

In Sanskrit, *dosha* means a system that is quick to change, that which has a fault. Doshas are of three types: Vata, Pitta and Kapha.

Vata has space and air as its dominant elements.

Pitta has fire as a dominant element.

Kapha has water and earth as its elements.

The ancient science of Ayurveda provides guidelines to identify our constitutional nature, which enables us to live wisely on the earth. The tridosha—Vata-Pitta-Kapha—are responsible for the arising of natural urges for preferences in foods: flavor, taste, et cetera. They are responsible for psychological processes, including emotions such as fear, anger, and greed and understanding, compassion, and love. The tridosha are the foundation of the existence of man. There is a ceaseless interaction between the internal and external environment, including cosmic forces (macrocosm) and internal forces (microcosm), which is governed by the tridosha.

The tridosha plays a very important role in the maintenance of health and longevity.

Vata—Governs all life functions. Closely related to pranic life energy

Pitta—Governs digestion and nutrition

Kapha—Maintains longevity

Ayurveda also indicates which type of yoga posture is suitable for each individual according to his constitution. If the percentage of these universal elements is known, we can do better to preserve our health. Hence, the universal elements serve as the foundation of all diagnosis and treatments in Ayurveda.

BODY CONSTITUTION

According to the Sankhya philosophy, matter or nature is composed of three modes: Sattva, Rajas, and Tamas. These three modes are the actual substances or ingredients of which the matter is constituted. Pure consciousness is devoid of these modes. The five gross elements (i.e., space, air, fire, water, and earth) exist in all matter, both organic and inorganic. All these elements exist within each individual and everything.

Deha means body constitution. Everything individual has a combination of the tridoshas, i.e., Vata, Pitta and Kapha, or a combination: Vata-Pitta, Pitta-Kapha, or Vata-Pitta-Kapha. To maintain good health, all these doshas should be in balance; out of balance means disease or ill health.

Mana is mental constitution. A person's dosha type is expressed emotionally as well. Vedic philosophy classifies human temperaments into three basic qualities: Sattva, Rajas, and Tamas.

Sattva: Neutral balanced, positive, cool, calm; disturbances can not affect this.

Rajas: This mode is activity, the factor responsible for change, with words to rearrange things and ideas.

Tamas: Binds things to their places; hates any alterations or renovations; orthodox in nature.

Out of the three modes Rajas and Tamas are known as Maha-Doshas and can cause problems to our bodies due to their tendency to negativity.

Sattva-is pure, with no question about the appearance of disease.

In order to have a harmonious life, it is suggested that we increase Sattva and keep a little of Rajas and Tamas to accommodate movement and rest. To help ourselves live a joyful and fulfilled life, we should become aware of our lifestyle and use tools such as breathing techniques, asanas, and meditation to calm and integrate the nervous system.

Sattva means good qualities of mind, Rajas means undesirable qualities of mind, and Tamas means bad qualities of mind. These three qualities of mind have a deep relation with the Ayurvedic system and treatments. Treatment of a Sattva person is maintained according to the nature of a Sattva person; similarly Rajas and Tamas persons are treated according to their natures. Though these qualities are transferred by parents to their children during fertilization, environment and diet play decisive roles in the formation of these three modes (Sattva, Rajas, Tamas).

Vata, Pitta, and Kapha are the three biological elements that constitute the structural and fundamental units of the body as a whole. Doshas, or the humors, act in the body in accordance with the five elements that are the basis of nature, as well as Ayurvedic theory of treatment.

Yoga therapy considers all eight limbs of yoga; it does not isolate physical aspect of yoga like asanas. According to the science of Ayurveda:, asanas are external medicine, while pranayama and meditation are internal medicine. According to this science of Ayurveda, our body should be appropriately nourished with appropriate food so that we can keep our doshas, or humors, in balance.

ANALYSIS OF DOSHAS AND THEIR CHARACTERISTICS

ANATOMY OF VATA

Vata, or air, means movement it is responsible for all mobility in all the directions. Vata molecules are light, minute, clear, rough, and dry. They quickly spread throughout the body and are cold in nature, causing diseases related to cold. Though it cannot be visualized in any form in the body, its presence can be proved by its actions. Vata is generally understood as the physical activity responsible for motion. It carries all the sensory impulses to their sensors and also maintains the efficiency of the sense organs.

FIVE TYPES OF VATA

Vata energy is divided into five types, called Vayus, or air.

1. **Prana** is located in the head and governs the chest, throat, heart, and sense organs, sneezing, and the swallowing of food.
2. **Udan**a resides in the chest and controls the nose, naval, throat, memory, and the capacity to walk.
3. **Vyana** is found in the heart and rapidly moves to the whole body. It controls the movements of the body, like walking and rising, the lowering of the body parts, and also opening and closing the eyes.
4. **Samana** digestive fire, is located near the navel. It works in the abdominal organs. It holds the food, absorbing nutrients and excreting wastes. It helps to digest food.
5. **Apan**a is located in the colon and regulates the waist, bladder, genitals, and thighs. It controls the downward movement of wastes (feces, urine), menstrual fluid, and the movement of a fetus.

CHARACTERISTICS OF VATA

- Light, thin-built. Finds gaining weight difficult
- Performs activities quickly; like walking or eating
- Irregular hunger and digestive; irregular sleeping habits
- Tendency to worry
- Mental or physical energy comes in bursts
- Tendency to overexert, gets tired easily
- Tendency to forget quickly
- Alteration in moods, unpredictable nature
- Under pressure grows excited and anxious
- Displays bursts of emotions that are short-lived and quickly forgotten

BASIC NATURE OF VATA

a. Changeability
b. Unpredictability
c. Variability

ANATOMY OF PITTA

Pitta represents energy in the body and is the combination of fire and water. Digestion entirely depends on Pitta (fire). The process of digestion in the gastrointestinal tract is done by means of various digestive and tissue enzymes, known as Pitta. It is hot, light, and clear. It is mobile, sour, and has a strong, foul smell. It moves on the principle of gravity, upward and downward. It increases heat and body temperatures, as well as appetite and thirst. It also maintains vision. All types of outside elements an individual takes in are transformed into inside elements of the body by Pitta. Pitta persons are prone to diseases of the digestive and metabolic systems.

FIVE TYPES OF PITTA

1) **Pachaka**: The gastrointestinal tract is the seat of Pachak Pitta. Pachaka (digestive enzymes) through digestion nourish the other four Pittas.

2) **Ranjak**: The main sites of this Pitta are the liver, spleen, stomach, and small intestines. It is represented by bile, enzymes, and bone marrow. Its junction is a synthesis of hemoglobin and imparts red color to the blood.

3) **Sodhaka**: The brain is the main site of Sodhaka Pitta. It is represented by the cellular enzymes of nerve cells.

4) **Alochak**: It exists in the eyes as light; i. e., worldly wisdom. It allows good processing of information, thereby leading to the maturity of comprehension.

5) **Bhrajak**: The skin is the main site of this Pitta. It keeps the skin warm and is responsible for its complexion.

CHARACTERISTICS OF PITTA

- Medium build; strength and endurance
- Sharp hunger and thirst, strong digestion; cannot skip meals
- Sharp intellect, precise speech, but often rude
- Enterprising character, likes challenges
- Tendency toward anger and irritability under stress
- Ambition, sharp wit, outspoken and argumentative
- Orderly management of money, energy, time, and action
- Impatient, demanding, perfectionist

THE BASIC NATURE OF PITTA

a) Intensity in all actions

ANATOMY OF KAPHA

It is derived from two basic physical elements: earth and water. Kapha molecules are heavy, stable, white in color, and have a salty taste. Kapha constitutes the body mass and is responsible for the shape and form of the body. The biological combination of solids and liquids in different proportions are responsible for varying structures and composition of tissues; body fluids, semen, blood, muscles, fat, bone marrow, and brain.

FIVE TYPES OF KAPHA

- **Kledak**: It is present in the stomach and intestines up to the colon. It dilutes the food taken and also helps digestion
- **Avalambak**: It is present in the chest. It constitutes the lung tissues. It also supports and gives strength to heart, lungs, and ribs.
- **Bodhak**: Present in the oral cavity and in the throat and is represented by saliva. It helps the tongue to appreciate taste.
- **Tarpak**: It is situated in the cranial cavity and is represented by cerebrospinal fluids.
- **Shleshak**: It represents the synovial fluid in the joints and provides nutrition to the ends of the bones.

CHARACTERISTICS OF KAPHA

- Solid, powerful build, great physical strength and endurance
- Tendency to obesity
- Slow digestion, mild hunger; tendency to oversleep
- Steady energy, slow and graceful in action
- Good retentive memory
- Affectionate, tolerant, forgiving, but possessive
- Takes a long time to arrive a decision

BASIC NATURE OF KAPHA

To be slow and relaxed

PHYSIOLOGY OF SAPTA DHATUS

DHATUS OR TISSUES

The second leg of the tripod of life, dhatus, or the tissues, are in fact products of digested food. Ayurveda places importance on the food we eat. Dhatus are made up of five elements, the Pancha mahabhutas. The predominant element in dhatus is earth, which gives them stability and prevents migration from one place to another.

The most important difference between dhatus and doshas is that dhatus perform functions under the fine-tuned control of the doshas. The food we eat is assimilated to form and replace the dhatus and, through them, the doshas, which in turn influence the function of the dhatus. In Sanskrit, *dhatus* means support. Ayurveda describes only seven major or functionally separate tissues.

The food consumed by us is how we nourish our bodies and minds. According to the science of Ayurveda, this process is completed in seven ways, or steps, one by one or simultaneously. These seven steps nourish the body by their activities and abilities and are as follows:

Rasa: It provides nourishment to the rest of the six dhatus and is the transporter of the body pleasure fluids.

Rakta: It provides energy to all five dhatus and gives color to the body.

Mamsa: It covers the body and gives movements to the body's muscular system.

Meda: It collects the energies and stores them for strength of the body.

Ashti: It supports the body and makes it stand upright.

Majja: It is responsible for love and nourishment, and its structure is smooth and soft; it fills the gaps in bones and is called marrow

Shukra: It is important for the reproductive capacities of a person.

These seven dhatus together hold up the body and provide strength for life. When these dhatus change, each tissue level is nourished. The Rasa Dhatus should be of a good quality.

TASTES

Tastes play a major role in Ayurveda. According to this science there are six tastes in every food, plant, and herb, et cetera. These play a vital role in the human body:

1. Sweet
2. Sour
3. Salty
4. Powerful
5. Bitter
6. Severe or sharp

These tastes have direct relation with the doshas, which in turn either aggravate or pacify the doshas. Also these tastes have a relation with the five universal elements as follows:

- Sweet, Powerful, and Sharp have a relationship with water
- Salty has a relationship with earth
- Sour has a relationship with fire
- Bitter has a relationship with air

MALA OR THE METABOLIC END PRODUCTS

This is the third leg of the tripod of life. Mala in Ayurveda is described as the waste products "of the body, like urine or feces. These waste products play an important function when inside our bodies. Academically, these waste products are interpreted as metabolic end products, which means that each cell is a living factory and under the influence of the doshas will produce chemicals, or mala, which in turn influence the function of the dhatus that manufacture them. The chemicals created on the spot by cells from their lifeline, oxygen, may be regarded as metabolic end products, or mala, of the cells. This illustrates the principles of Ayurveda: keep all the legs of the tripod—dosha, dhatus, and mala—healthy, and you will not face disease".

THE DRIVING FORCE, AGNI

According to the ancient Ayurvedic physician Charaka, "Agni is responsible for life, the body, tissues, strength, and the complexion of a person." Agni in the Veda is always presented in the double aspect of force and light. He is the divine power that builds up the world's power, which acts always with a perfect knowledge. It is said that "Agni is the immortal in mortals, the energy through which they do their work in him. Because Agni is born in the body of a human, he is turned as his son. Agni grows in the human body and manifests his power." (RigVeda)

Agni is the fire that cooks or digests the food. Agni, according to Ayurveda, influences all the processes whether in the tissues or stomach or in the elements.

SOME TREATMENTS OF DISEASE: SAMPRAPTI

According to the Sankhya philosophy, transcending the modes or the gunas in a human body can lead us to remove the dhuka, or suffering, and that can be attained through the practice of yoga asanas, pranyayama, and meditation, which is contemplation, or by introspection.

Samprapti is the result of accumulation of the doshas in:

Vata: colon
Pitta: small intestine
Kapha: stomach

Due to dietary factors, this initial stage is a starting place for disease.

Aggravation: where doshas are not in their normal site

Overflow: doshas disperse to new sites

Relocation: disturbances move to different sites

Manifestation: the disease becomes evident

Chronic: unrecoverable stage

The basic of Ayurvedic treatment is a process of purification. The accumulation of toxic substances, years of poor diet, weak digestion, incomplete elimination of waste matter, improper sleep, and, above all, stress leads to the imbalance of the tridoshas, which becomes the cause of diseases.

According to Ayurveda:

Shamana Chikitsa: Treats and manages diseases that have already manifested with the help of herbs and mineral products and also by other medicines.

Shodana Chikitsa: Is based on an internal process of purification used to cure and prevent diseases. This purification process is mainly done in three stages: pre-purification, main, and post-purification. Yoga philosophy is an approach to a disciplined way of life for purification and for spiritual well-being and is a righteous way to bring about the Ayurvedic healing. Constitutions do not change, but every individual has a body, mind, and soul unlike that of any other. Different combinations of doshas provide information on our metabolic tendencies, which must remain in balance, and the foundation is to practice prescribed yoga asanas and the internal yogas.

ASANAS FOR DIFFERENT TYPES OF BODY CONSTITUTIONS

ASANAS USEFUL FOR BALANCING VATA

(Visudha, Anhata Chakra)

Lotus pose (Padmasana)
Tree pose (Trikonasana)
Slow sun salutations (Surya Namasakar)
Plow pose (Halasana)
Knee to chest (Muktasana)
Shoulder stand (Sarvangasana)
Cobra pose (Bhujangasana)
Bow pose (Dhanurasana)
Head down (yogins sealing posture)
Corpse pose (Savasana)
Slow grounding practice (Garudasana)

Vata should practice slowly and deliberately. Vata types are connected to air and space, so they are similar to the wind—dry, cool, and capable of fast, unpredictable movement and thought.

When Vata gets out of control, there is tendency toward gas and stomachache.

Full yogic breath exercise is necessary, also deep concentration (meditation) Vatas benefit from jasmine and rose.

ASANAS USEFUL FOR BALANCING PITTA

(Manipura, Svadhisthana)

Level 1

Sun Salutation (Surya Namaskar)

Cobra (Bhujangasana)
Forward bend (Paschimottasana)
Triangular Pose (Trikonasana)
Twist (Matsyendrasana)
Boat pose (Navasana)
Fish pose (matsyasana)
Corpse pose(Savasana)

Level 2

Shoulder to head (Sarvangasana)
Plow pose (Halasana)

For Pitta, the adoption of a relaxed, non-hurried, gentle, and patient attitude to one's Sadhna will have a positive effect. Choose cooling pranayama, shitali pranyayama, full yogic breath, and quiet breathing (i.e., deep meditation)

Pitta need to relax and avoid overheating and are aligned with fire, influenced by fire, and act with intense determination. When Pitta flares, it will spawn anger and irritability. A spirit of calming and cooling is important.

ASANAS USEFUL FOR BALANCING KAPHA

(Muladhara, Svadhisthana)

Triangle pose (Trikonasana)
Backward bend (Bhujangasana)
Plow pose (Halasana)
Forward bend (Pascimotasana)
Fish pose (Matsyeasana)
Inverted pose (Sarvangasana)
Bow pose (Dhanurasana)
Head knee pose (Pavan Muktasana)

Cobra pose (Bhujangasana)
Boat pose (Navasana)
The Half Moon (Ardha chandrasana)
Strong Sun Salutations (Surya Namaskara)

Pranayama Kapalbati, Bastrika, and meditation are recommended. Kapha predominates in inertia and lethargy; lack of motivation keeps them from moving forward.

Kapha types often tend to suffer from asthma and extra mucus. Sprinkles of scented water help kaphas to relax.

AYURVEDIC AND YOGIC DIET FOR WELL-BEING

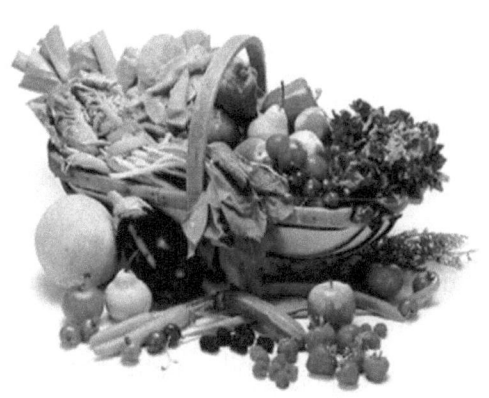

Ayurvedic and Yogic diet

In the Vedas we read that "The fountain for all actions is the perfection of the body." And further, "One who is weak cannot have experience of the soul." Thus the body is the fountain for the evolution of each individual. The aim of yoga and Ayurveda is almost the same; both are concerned with our well-being. According to the Ayurvedic belief, choosing what to eat depends not only on what suits your dosha but also on some complex factors like: Season, location, and one's taste. Food is agreeable to different people according to their innate dispositions, like Sattavika, Rajasika, or Tamasika. If a man's diet is pure, his mind will be pure. According to Upanishad, "Purity of mind follows from the purity of diet." And purity of thought and feelings, of faith and other qualities like actions depend on purity of mind. The foods are also of the types Sattvika, Rajasika, and Tamasika.

Sattavika-types of foods include: most vegetables, clarified butter, fruit, legumes, whole grain, sweets, milk products and skimmed milk, sunflower seeds, herbs, and teas.

Rajaskida-types of foods include those that are bitter, acid, salty, spicy, overhot, dry, burning, including coffee.

Tamasida-types of foods include: half-cooked, half-ripe, insipid, putrid, polluted, impure meat, and garlic; also intoxicants, such as spirituous liquor.

According to the Vedic traditions there are two categories: 1) Foods for a student of yoga. 2) Foods that may be eaten, though they are declined by the Vedic traditions.

FORBIDDEN FOODS

    A. He shall not eat food which has been bought or obtained ready-prepared in the market.

    B. Nor shall he eat flavored food bought in the market.

    C. Prepared food which has stood for a night must neither be eaten nor drunk.

    D. Nor should prepared food that has turned sour be used in anyway.

    E. Substances which have turned sour without being mixed with anything else are to be avoided.

    F. All intoxicating drinks are forbidden.

G. Foods mixed herbs which serve for preparing intoxicating liquors must not be taken.

H. Red garlic, onion, and leeks must be avoided.

I. Food given unwillingly by a holy man ought not to be eaten.

ABOUT THE AUTHOR

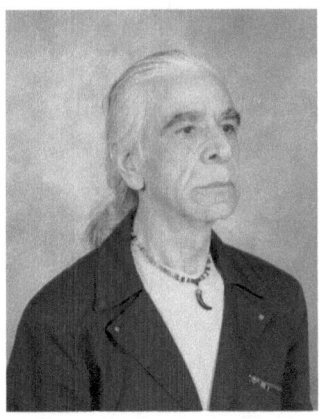

Lalit Kilam was born and raised in the mountainous region of the Himalayas. He received a master's degree in engineering at one of the prestigious universities in Europe. He has been servicing computers and connecting the masses by providing Internet services via high speed and wireless broadband in various countries. He has traveled extensively and has knowledge of several prominent languages.

Because of years of study and experience, he is able to provide the groundwork for a Western understanding of yoga, in theory and in practice, from its earliest roots in the Vedas. He is the founder of the Vedic Yoga Center in Lloydminster, Sk.

A born Brahmin who has extensively studied the natural sciences and ancient Eastern and Western philosophies, he realized the scientific nature underlying the philosophy of yoga, its practical dimensions, and its implications in daily life as an approach toward the betterment of human life. He believes yoga contributes to the ancient Eastern and Western philosophies can be made comprehensible to scholars and common people alike. He ardently believes that yoga is a mantra for spiritual education and enlightenment and a path to freedom. According to him, yoga is not something you have to train for or a skill you want to add; it is a mantra—something you naturally are, your internal realm.

His previous literary works include *Existence and Beyond, Yoga Practices, Existence and Yoga,* and *Philosophy of Yoga.* He also has published numerous articles in the arts journals and newspapers.

**Yoga is a Mantra . . . It is just a reminder to
return home, what is natural to you.**

NOTES

i   Schopenhauer Arthur, "The World as Idea." In *Philosophy of Recent Times vol 1*, ed. Hartman B. James (New York: McGraw Hill Book Company), p. 83-84.

ii   *Vivekananda*, vol. 2., p. 442.

iii   Abhedananda Swami, *The Vedanta Philosophy*, (rpt.Calcutta: Ramkrishna Math, 1993), p. 13.

iv   Swami Rama, *Choosing a Path*. Himalayan International Institute of Yoga Science and Philosophy of the U.S.A.,1996, p.178.

INDEX

www.ingramcontent.com/pod-product-compliance
Lightning Source LLC
Chambersburg PA
CBHW061312280526
45784CB00002B/967